THE FORMULA

THE
FORMULA

Who Gets Sick, Who Gets Well,
Who Is Happy, Who Is Unhappy,
and Why

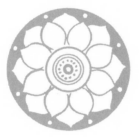

VERNON M. SYLVEST, M.D.

THE FORMULA:
Who Gets Sick, Who Gets Well,
Who Is Happy, Who Is Unhappy and Why.

© 1996 VERNON M. SYLVEST, M.D.

© United States Copyright, 1999
Sunstar Publishing, Ltd.
204 South 20th Street
Fairfield, Iowa 52556

Cover Design: Amanda Collett
Text Design and Production Coordination
by Laura Cruger Fox, Richmond Virginia.

Library of Congress Catalog Card Number: 99-61228
ISBN: 1-887472-65-7

First Printing, 1999
Printed in the U.S.A.

Readers interested in obtaining further information on the subject
matter of this book are invited to correspond with
The Secretary, Sunstar Publishing, Ltd.
204 South 20th Street, Fairfield, Iowa 52556

*This book is dedicated
to you.*

CONTENTS

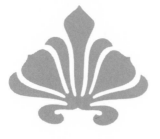

ACKNOWLEDGEMENTS

M any teachers have made the writing of this book possible. They include every individual who has participated in my life directly or indirectly. The list is obviously too long to recount here. Some I have known personally, others I have known through their work. They are all important, although some stand out now as I reflect on the history behind the making of this book. These include the late Helen Schucman and William Thetford, whose willingness (along with others) brought us *A Course in Miracles* (ACIM)[17] which has had a tremendous impact on my life; Levi Dowling, whose dedication and inspiration brought us the clear message of *The Aquarian Gospel of Jesus the Christ* (Aq.G.)[23]; Starr Daily, who at one time was Al Capone's chief henchman, but who through willingness was open to receive a revelation experience that led to his own healing and learning. Daily's book, *Release*,[18] was of special value to me. Also included is Dr. George Ritchie, who was willing to share the message of his near-death experience in his book *Return from Tomorrow*[94] and with me in person. It was Raymond Moody's association with Dr. Ritchie as a psychiatric resident that inspired Dr. Moody to do the pioneer near-death study published in *Reflections on Life After Life*.[65] I am grateful to Margaret Kean, whose near-death revelation led her into healing work, which so influenced my life, and to Nancy Clark, whose revelation experience led to her healing work and loving, helpful support. They were both able to confirm much of what I had been learning from my own experience.

I also extend my gratitude to the many men and women of science whose work has brought our culture to a point where it is possible to integrate spiritual teachings and scientific information toward greater understanding of our true nature, and to the students and teachers of modern psychology for revealing unseen dynamics of consciousness so we can better understand the blocks to our experience of our true nature.

On a more personal note, I extend my heartfelt gratitude to my mother and father, Vera and Edwin. Their devotion and perseverance, which laid the foundation for me, came from their own experience of love and from the teachings of the Bible, which they spoon-fed (and at times force-fed) me. Thanks go to orthodox Christianity, for pre-serving the history of Jesus and his teachings through the ages. Although not clearly understood or delivered, these teachings supplied the toe-hold that resulted in my choosing to persevere and the spring-board that led to my success.

Thanks also to the many family members—grandparents, aunts, uncles, cousins and brother—who left their marks of love, which I have never forgotten. Special thanks go to my brother, Ed, for being such an excellent role-model during my childhood. One day in the sixth grade while I was being admonished by the school principal for my angry behavior, I was asked, "Why don't you be nice like your brother?" For some reason, probably because of the degree of trouble I thought I was in (in those days of corporal punishment, a trip to the principal's office was no trifling matter), I decided to do it. It was a good choice.

To my three daughters, Tasha, Rebecca and Vivian, I extend my deep gratitude for their continued devotion, even during the depths of my despair, which so affected them, and to Juanita, my former wife, for giving birth to them and for her integrity and desire for truth that led to forgiveness and clear friendship. I also extend gratitude to Sharon for the role she agreed to play in our lives, which for me was a moulding experience.

I extend my deep gratitude to my wife, Anne, who has shared herself with me from the wholeness that she is. Together we have learned that it is possible for couples to have happy, long-term relationships. Thanks go to her for her support in this work and to her family, which is now also part of my family, for accepting me with love.

And finally, my deep gratitude goes to the father-and-daughter team, George Cruger (editing) and Laura Cruger Fox (text design and production coordination), and to the Sunstar staff including Rodney Charles (publisher) and Elizabeth Pasco (text design) whose work and support helped make this book possible.

INTRODUCTION

Ten years ago I was in a neighbor's living room explaining to her a small bit of what I had learned over the preceding two years when she looked at me with great curiosity and asked, "Vernon, are you writing a book?" It was then that I knew I would. I didn't know it would take ten years—ten years not in the writing but in the making. This book describes some of my life experiences, how they led to disease and the learning that led to recovery. As my learning has brought me healing and joy, it is my hope that this book will bring similar healing and joy to your life and the lives of others you will touch in your own experiences.

Although I have journeyed from the brink of death and emotional disaster to health, success and happiness, I am not so arrogant as to claim that my pain was worse than yours. Each person's pain is the worst for him or her. I have chosen not to include all of the details of my personal hell, but it took me to the depths of emotional and physical pain, as deep as anyone can descend and still be alive. That journey was not one that I consciously chose, but through my willingness to learn it has brought me much understanding of the pain of others and the wisdom to help guide others out of their pain. While I was suffering, I was told the future would be good. I did not believe that advice; so it came as little comfort. Yet for some reason, which I will not analyze here, I did persevere, and now I am in that future. It is good. Miracles do happen, and they are waiting to happen to you. This book will help you to become miracle-ready.

One of the things that helped me become ready was the scientific information now available and to which I was surely led. It opened the door to understanding and to a new level of scientific experience for me. This information has been extremely useful in my efforts to help others, as well. In the West we have placed science on the pedestal of leadership and have allowed social and economic pressures to decide who the valid scientists are. However, in the experience of the human spirit the true pioneers have come forth to perform. When you are ready and willing, that help will be there for you, just as this book is in your hands now.

It is now possible for you to know what you need to know to be well and happy. It is now possible to live as a whole, fully integrated individual, free of the shackles of not knowing who you are.

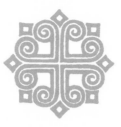

Chapter 1

ATTEMPT AT SELF DISCOVERY

Humankind has experienced disease, strife and unhappiness throughout its history. Why? Is it our nature to be constantly threatened by pain and suffering? What is our nature? Who are we that this should happen?

Our culture spends a tremendous amount of money, time and effort to answer this question. In the sciences of chemistry, physics and biology, we are spending billions on research. Social scientists in a variety of fields are in search of the answer. Psychologists, too. Theologians are spending their lives attempting to answer this question. Something is driving us, and that something is the sense that if we discover who we are, we can make our circumstances better, and we will be happier. This intuitive sense exists within everyone. Even as a young lad I had the feeling that if I knew who I was, I would have the secret to happiness. I knew at the age of three that I wasn't always happy, and the older I got the more aware I was that I was unhappy. Because my unhappiness seemed to be increasing, my efforts to discover who I was intensified.

Since I thought I was a physical body, I developed an avid interest in biology. The subject piqued my curiosity with the anticipation of discovery. Thus I pursued biology in high school and college. This interest led to the study of medicine, which allowed for an in-depth study of human biology. It served well my attempt at self discovery because not only was I a healthy body, but sometimes I was also a sick body. What better way to study myself, I thought, than to dissect a human body, look at it under the microscope, examine it chemically and study its physiology and pathology.

But I didn't limit my search to the study of the body. I was also aware that I had a mind, so I pursued its study as well. Even as a lad in middle school I attempted to satisfy my curiosity by reading my father's psychology books. But this didn't help matters. His books were all on abnormal psychology, and I came away frightened that I also might be abnormal. I thought I recognized myself in some of the neuroses that were described.

I also studied theology. My father had a doctorate in theology, so I had a ready tutor. Yet I observed that he was stoically unhappy. I pursued this area in college, but any answer I found always led to another question, until a final leap of faith was required. But it was a leap that I was unable to make. Besides, many of my colleagues who said they had made that leap did not impress me as being happy.

I did find a few people, however, who, through personal experience independent of study, had become happier than most. This was a curiosity to me, and I sought out these people. Listening to them share their experiences, however, did not lead to any immediate revelation, although I filed this information away for later use.

In medical school I also had the required opportunity to study the mind through psychiatry, which was mostly Freudian in orientation, but this only led to more confusion. My conclusion at that time, based on my limited exposure, was that psychiatrists were the most confused of all and had been attracted to psychiatry in an attempt to figure out what was wrong with themselves. In fact, just as I was, they were attempting to discover who they were.

I recall a patient to whom I was assigned in the psychiatric outpatient clinic who was suffering from severe depression. As she explained her life situation—how her husband had left her and her children had deserted her, leaving her with no family or friends—I found myself also becoming depressed. I realized I had nothing to offer her except a prescription for antidepressants, which I doubted would do little more than dull her pain. However, I did not prescribe any for myself, even though I left the encounter also depressed. I tried to forget her and what her experience implied about myself by becoming distracted with other activities.

I gave up on the study of the mind, focusing my attention exclusively on molecular medicine. I had planned to become an internist since this specialty dealt with "reality" (the physical body) and encompassed most aspects of the adult body's experience. This would allow me to continue to seek the solution to the mystery of my nature.

This endeavor did not fare well. If what I was discovering represented who I was, I did not like what I was finding. Most of my training was in the acute-care hospital setting, where most of the patients were seriously ill. The majority came to the internist with chronic diseases that were progressive in nature. It seemed as if 80% of the patients continued to deteriorate. I was able only to delay the deterioration and help make the patients more comfortable until their inevitable demise. In some cases, however, they seemed to be made worse by therapy. For me, the study and practice of internal medicine was depressing and laced with futility.

This frustration led to a search for another specialty. Pathology had been my favorite area of study in medical school. The word pathology literally means the study of disease. It is the science of medicine. It touches all specialties and is the basis for understanding their practices. Thus pathology seemed to offer the ultimate approach to understanding myself, for it dealt most directly with the anatomical and molecular structure and function of the body. Furthermore, as a specialty it avoided some of the frustration of internal medicine. For one thing, the pathologist is always successful. He can put a name on the disease or anatomical finding and thus make a diagnosis. It is ultimately the internist who must deal with the likelihood of not being able to offer a cure.

The practice of pathology, however, did not lead me to my goal of self discovery. I dissected many hearts but did not find a feeling. I dissected and studied many brains but did not find a thought. I learned a lot about sickness and dead bodies, and what I discovered was at best discouraging. The worst experiences came not from the dead bodies but from the dying ones. In the hospital I saw people with shriveled-up bodies and non-functioning or poorly functioning brains experiencing a lot of pain. I realized they had once been in their prime, as I should have been then. But there they were, in terminal misery. Why? What was it all about? Life seemed like some sort of cruel practical joke.

My experience of self discovery was not leading to happy results. It was actually leading to depression.

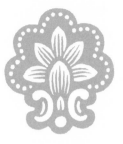

Chapter 2

ATTEMPT AT SELF CREATION

In the absence of knowing who I was, I was also involved in another process, that of creating myself. It was not enough simply to exist. I knew that I was Vernon Sylvest, the son of Vera and Edwin Sylvest, and a male human being. But that was not good enough. I needed other standards by which to define myself. What I was seeking was a definition of self as worthy, important and respected, for I secretly suspected that I might not be worthy or respectable. This perception was associated with feelings of guilt, which led to fear, both of which are obviously the antithesis of happiness. If I could become what others approved, that approval would define me as worthy. Then, I thought, I would be happy.

In the absence of knowing who we are, self definition or self creation will always be attempted to some degree. After having spent a good portion of my adult life attempting to create myself, I can now say that it cannot be done. It will always lead to failure and disappointment. We cannot create ourselves because we have already been created. However, the attempt to do so is the basis of much commercial activity and spawns commercial enterprises costing billions of dollars. Much more money is spent on creating ourselves than on discovering ourselves.

We attempt to create ourselves according to the standards given to us by whomever we learn to respect or on whom we have been taught to depend. In other words, what is good and worthwhile to us will be determined most immediately by our family and peers and then by our culture generally. We learn that if we are a certain way we will be "somebody."

My father was well educated; he had a doctorate in theology and a master's degree in psychology. Both of my parents often spoke of his accomplishments and the value of education. They also spoke somewhat disparagingly about those who had not pursued higher education. It was a given that I must go to college and beyond. Thus I obtained an undergraduate degree with all the scholastic honors available. I also obtained a professional degree in medicine, again with all the scholastic honors that could be acquired, including finishing first in my class. Then there was post-doctoral training in pathology so that I could be a specialist. However, complete happiness still eluded me. There was always something more that I had to accomplish in order to escape the feeling of self-doubt. That feeling, of course, is guilt. Frequently it is experienced simply as boredom. Boredom is actually a subtle form of depression, the first hint of the lack of joy caused by repressed guilt.

My father was also a Methodist minister; thus I was well indoctrinated into the moral principles of a virtuous life. To be morally correct was to be worthy. So I led a disciplined, stringent, moral life. My adolescent and young adult life would not make very interesting pop reading, although my imagination would have made a novel of some notoriety.

To be validated by other people was all-important. To have people willing to be my friends would indicate that I must be "okay." Thus an active social life was important. But most important was to have a wife—someone to love me more than anyone else, so much so that she would commit the rest of her life to me and have my children. This was an early goal of mine. Since I was not sure of my own value, as a college sophomore and fraternity man I dated a freshman who because of her intellectual abilities had skipped her senior year in high school and had started college at age sixteen. This served two purposes. Having a smart girlfriend would validate my worthiness, but since she was so young and new to the college scene I could fool her into thinking I was somebody great. I succeeded, and she agreed to marry me after my junior year.

Second to having a woman commit to me as a wife would be to have children who would dote on me. Such validation would be a great source of happiness. From my point of view, having girls would be even better, for they would dote more on the father than sons would. We had three daughters.

In addition, it was important for me to be physically strong, virile and successfully competitive. This need was satisfied through athletics. This activity helped in high school, although happiness still eluded me. However, since scholastic accomplishments had been stressed in my family, I sacrificed athletics for scholarship in college. Yet any show of physical strength still remained an important source of personal pride.

Then, of course, there were money and material things. I was not immune to these cultural influences in spite of my strict puritanical background. As a minister's family, we were respected but poor. However, my parents' worrying about money did not teach me that poverty was virtuous. Thus I looked forward to the economic advantage of a medical career.

Chapter 3

FAILURE

It would seem that I had it all: advanced education, a respected profession and money; wife, children and friends; a strong, virile body and good morals. Yet it was not enough. My seemingly successful attempt to create myself was not successful because I was not happy. For one thing, there were constant reminders all around me that I could lose everything.

I was a respected pathologist in my community but was not fulfilled. There were more goals to be achieved. I was not at that time the director of the laboratory. Nor was I nationally known. However, national recognition would have required the sacrifice of my family and social life, and this I was not willing to do. I now know that had I achieved those goals, it still would not have been enough.

I was married to a smart, attractive wife, but once I got her, I simply projected my own feelings of inadequacy onto her. Because she was mine, I felt there must be something wrong with her. Besides, once we were married it seemed to me that her commitment was out of obligation and not voluntary. I missed the surge of satisfaction brought on by someone new and different saying I was okay. In addition, as I became familiar with her self doubts, I began to question her value in defining my worth.

Another more subtle undermining factor was also in operation. Unconsciously I "knew" that I was using her to define myself, taking from her to make myself whole but giving little in return. This activity was associated with repressed guilt. Her presence stirred up this feeling, which was immediately translated into anger toward her. Thus I frequently found myself irritated without reasonable cause, for instance by the way she combed her hair, how she dressed or what she said or did. And she was going through the same dynamic with me. This did not make for a happy marriage, but I was morally trapped and did the best I could to fulfill my obligation.

The children were truly a source of joy, but because of my need for professional success and my desire to spend less time with my wife, I spent less time in family activities.

Eventually things began to get worse. My wife, fed up with what she called a "charade of a marriage," left. At first that seemed like a good deal. Because of her desire to pursue an advanced education and career, she chose to leave the children with me, making the deal seem even better. I was excited at the prospect of finding a better woman to take her place. But there was a problem. I was attempting to create myself by being morally correct, which required an intact family. By my own standards divorce was out of the question, but since my wife was determined, it was out of my hands. I felt immoral, and the fact that I was glad that she was leaving worsened my guilt, making it impossible for me to enjoy my new "happy" situation.

So two of the five parameters by which I had been measuring myself were gone—family and morals. I had my profession, but that wasn't enough. My body was still strong and the material aspects of my world were adequate, but it was a world without happiness. I was acutely depressed.

On April 10, 1977, I lost another defining parameter. It happened on a Sunday, ironically. Within a few hours, I went from robust health to an invalid in severe pain. I awoke with a strange pain in the middle of my back the likes of which I had never experienced. The back pain gradually went away during the morning, but later that afternoon pain developed in my right foot, increasing to a degree greater than I had ever experienced in my life. I could walk only with crutches. After a few days of examination and laboratory tests I received probably the most depressing news I had ever heard. I was told I had a form of chronic arthritis that was considered incurable. It was hoped that the disease could be controlled with medications, but the most effective drug was potentially fatal. The diagnosis was made conclusive by the discovery of an abnormal tissue antigen in my white blood cells. I had a genetic marker for this form of arthritis. The disease was not controlled by drugs, and over the next few weeks it progressed, marching through multiple joints and tissues.

I was so depressed at this point that my medical colleagues suggested that I seek psychiatric help. Thus began my journey into the experience of myself as a sick, chronically depressed person and a patient of traditional medicine and psychotherapy. In fact, I had been chronically depressed most of my life, but now I was no longer able to run from the feelings, although I still desperately tried.

I sought a substitute family in another woman, but try as I might the now-unrepressed feelings of guilt blocked my efforts. I sought physical health through all the traditional medical remedies known for my disease, but without relief. In spite of my disease, I pursued my career in pathology with increased activity, to the extent that I was able. I also pursued material happiness by investing in a variety of get-rich-quick schemes. I devoted much time to trying to be both mother and father to my daughters. I continued to spar emotionally with my ex-wife in an attempt to absolve myself of feelings of guilt. As before, none of it worked. My disease progressed. I was in constant pain. And my depression progressed until it became so severe that in the summer of 1981 I began to experiment with a new tri-cyclic antidepressant. The side effects of this seemed to further destroy my body.

My fear and depression were so intense that for three months I was unable to sleep. Sleeping pills seemed to have no effect. To physically move my body was like moving lead. I was experiencing the psychomotor retardation of depression. The simplest task required major effort and was associated with dread. Social interaction became a chore, and I avoided it as much as possible. At work I performed like a rusty robot in need of a grease job.

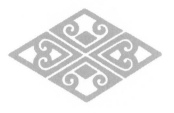

Chapter 4

SURRENDER AND SUCCESS

Death would have been welcomed, and I even planned several schemes of suicide. But I had just renewed my life-insurance policy and had another six months to go on the two-year waiting period for payment for suicide. Then my physical condition seemed to start cooperating with my desire. I developed cardiac arrhythmias, which required drug therapy. If I took enough of the drug it would cause a fatal arrhythmia and no one would suspect the truth. I carried enough of the medication with me in my briefcase to do the job in case things became totally unbearable.

Yet something held me back: my kids, a sense of responsibility and a faint thread of hope. That thread lay in my religious background from childhood. I knew it would take a miracle for me to be well and happy again. Because my state of mind was no longer logical, I began to hope that miracles were possible. So I began to pray and asked others to pray for me, from a charismatic minister who spoke in tongues to an Episcopal minister who used forms of prayer with which I was more familiar. My dear Uncle Ralph, one of my few relatives in the area outside of my immediate family, in his ever-patient love, never lost hope for me. Once a month, every second Sunday, he brought me to the Order of Saint Luke's healing service at the Episcopal church he attended. There, Rev. Rufus Womble prayed for and with me many times.

Words cannot convey the magnitude of what followed. Within nine months I was free of a disease that I had thought was incurable, and was well on the road to complete emotional recovery. The miracle did happen, although not as fast as I would have liked. There were a few more harrowing experiences awaiting me in the process, as well as some quite phenomenal experiences, which I am now more fully able to understand and appreciate.

Two of the more significant experiences follow. Shortly after the beginning of my prayer therapy a neighbor gave me a book entitled *Prison to Praise*[10] by Merlin Carothers, a minister. As a young adult Carothers had a crisis that led to his surrender and dramatic transformation. This led to a ministry in which he witnessed dramatic healing in some of those for whom he prayed. In my illogical state of mind, I hoped that he would pray for me and that I would experience an immediate healing. I heard that he was speaking in Augusta, Georgia, which is not too far away from my home in Richmond, Virginia. In my sickened state it was not an easy journey. When I arrived I spent most of the time in bed in the hotel. But I managed to make it to the coliseum where he was to speak. Amazingly, he began his sermon by describing a pathologist performing an autopsy. His description was quite detailed and more appropriate for pathology students than for the audience he was addressing. I realized that something significant was occurring. I was aware of Carl Jung's concept of synchronicity.[50] I was a pathologist, and Rev. Carothers was describing an autopsy just as I would have performed it; but he didn't know I was in the audience. He didn't know me at all.

In describing the autopsy, Rev. Carothers created an analogy. As we dissect the body to understand the physical changes that seem to cause disease, so must we also dissect our spiritual nature to understand the disturbance that is the real cause of disease. Although I registered this sermon as a significant event, I was too miserable to focus on the message at the time. I was looking for an instant cure. After the sermon Rev. Carothers did not have a healing service. I had to chase him out the back door to get a word with him. He seemed hurried and reluctant to talk to me, and even more reluctant to pray for me. But I insisted, and he did. Nothing happened. He had probably known that it wouldn't, thus the reluctance. I flew home as sick as I had been when I left. Disappointed, I quickly forgot about his sermon.

Finally in the early spring of 1982 I decided to take another stab at traditional medicine. I traveled to Duke Medical Center in Durham, North Carolina, to see what they could do for me. There I had another significant encounter, but not in the realm of medical therapy. At the time of my arrival a local television show featured Dr. Alan Whanger, who described his research on the Shroud of Turin. I listened with amazement as Dr. Whanger described evidence that seemed to indicate that the Shroud was the real burial cloth of Jesus and that it contained a miraculous image that seemed to have been caused by an energy release that may have been associated with a resurrection process. He was a psychiatrist at Duke Medical Center, so I sought him out. Dr. Whanger pointed me to the literature pertaining to recent research done on the Shroud.[39, 118] In the fall of 1978, forty American scientists went to Turin, a city in northern Italy, to study the cloth with modern instrumentation. After examining their data with as much objectivity as I could muster, it seemed to me that the only logical conclusion was that the cloth was just what the faithful said it was. (At that time I did not have the carbon dating data to deal with.)*

---

* I have subsequently evaluated the carbon dating information on the Shroud and discussed it with Dr. Whanger, who has been in communication with the other original scientists. Their conclusion, and mine as well, is that the carbon dating was a total fiasco and its information useless. The problem lies in the contamination of the cloth as it was handled throughout the centuries, its scorching and the method of sampling. It may take a few more attempts before useful information is obtained.

My encounter with the Shroud stimulated a greater interest in studying the teachings of Jesus. I also studied all forms of Christianity. This interest spilled over to a study of all the world's religions. What I found also stimulated my interest in science at a deeper level. I developed a compulsion to study the most recent concepts of modern physics. As in my encounters with Merlin Carothers and Dr. Whanger, further synchronicities led to other encounters of both a scientific and a spiritual or mystical nature to satisfy my compulsion. In the process I began to have my own experiences of inner knowing. As a result of this new approach and a willingness to see things differently, I discovered the answer to the unanswerable question: I discovered who I was. I discovered why I got sick. I discovered how to get well and stay well.

Some two years later as I was sharing my experience in a talk I was giving in a local church, it suddenly dawned on me that I had done exactly what Rev. Carothers had said to do. I had dissected my spiritual nature and understood the cause of my illness, and I had made the appropriate changes and gotten well.

What I changed was my attitude. The perceptions we hold and their accompanying emotions define our attitudes. My attitude changed from one of fear and guilt to one of innocence, trust and the willingness to love everyone, including myself.

Part of my lesson was realizing the effect my attitude had on others. People began to take comfort in my presence and would come to me "out of the blue" to seek counsel. Some felt comfortable enough with me to ask for help dealing with their physical pain. I found that if I touched them with the willingness to love and the intent to relieve their pain, their pain would in most cases go away. To my further amazement I found that I could do needle biopsies on patients without causing pain and, in many cases, without the usual bleeding. I would ask them after I finished, "Are you okay?" The frequent response would be, "Have you done it yet?"

I found that I could enhance this effect with focused intent over distance and have it work without the knowledge of the recipient. I first discovered this ability with children. In the check-out line of a local supermarket a mother and her two-year-old child were standing six feet ahead of me. The child was having a tantrum. He wanted this, then that, and in response to his mother's refusal he wailed loudly. My first reaction was a feeling of irritation, but I chose to let the feeling go and see the situation another way. I tried to understand the frustration the boy was feeling. I looked at him with the intent to love him, cradling him mentally in an attitude of prayer. In about two minutes the boy became calm and silent. He turned to look at me with amazement. Apparently he intuitively felt something coming from me. But I had failed to focus this energy of love on the mother. Although the boy was now quiet, she was still in the past, and as they left the store she grabbed the boy's hand in anger and jerked him away. The child began to cry again.

At the time I made this discovery, I was doing a lot of traveling, so I began to focus on comforting infants in airport terminals and airplanes. I found that I could almost always mentally comfort a crying infant so that it was at peace within a few seconds to less than two minutes. Sometimes the child would stop in mid-cry. In the past, I had avoided infants in close places, particularly on planes because they usually fretted noisily through the pressure changes. On one occasion I successfully offered silent comfort to an infant in the boarding area of the terminal. Then to my consternation I found myself seated face-to-face with the child. She was in her mother's lap and the front seat of the passenger section had been turned to face the rear. Hoping for a silent ride, I focused on the child the entire journey with the intent to love. The child did not utter a sound and for most of the journey stared at me wide-eyed.

I began to use this technique on patients who came to the hospital laboratory where I worked. The first experience was unplanned. An elderly woman was being wheeled into the waiting room where she was to wait for her blood to be drawn for admission lab work. As she began to lose her composure and break down in tears, I stood in the secretarial area on the other side of the glass from her. I paused, looked at the floor, offered a prayer of love and then looked at her for a moment, mentally wrapping her in love. I observed a dramatic, instant transformation as she was obviously comforted. My first experiences with this phenomenon astounded me. I have since become more used to the dramatic effect of focused love, although to see it in action is always gratifying. However, free will operates. We cannot force this comfort on others, although in my experience approximately 80% of both children and adults do respond.

The immediate benefit of love extended is not limited to the one who accepts it. The one who gives also receives. Once I was walking through a busy shopping mall feeling a sense of love and compassion for everyone. Strangers would smile and speak to me. When I went into a store to look at area rugs, the clerk was taking inventory and at first didn't appear to want to be bothered. I looked around on my own, and when I was ready to be helped I just stood there patiently, focusing love on the clerk. He left his inventory almost immediately and came over to me and quite graciously offered me the aid I needed. His mood improved steadily as he waited on me. I selected the small rug I wanted and took it to the check-out counter. One person was in front of me. I stood there only a moment when the original clerk came over to me some distance from his work area and told me that he would check me out so I wouldn't have to wait. It was clear to me that this was not his usual duty. Normally he would have been spending this time on the inventory.

Such experiences fueled my scientific curiosity. I extended my pursuit of quantum physics to include the physics of consciousness. This led to the understanding that thoughts and emotions are non-local, powerfully effective energy. My more practical curiosity was fueled as well. So when I heard there was a nurse in the area teaching a course in healing-touch therapy, I enrolled. My intent was to listen and observe for conceptual understanding but not to actively participate. After all, I was a pathologist, not a healing-touch therapist. In addition to the class work, the students were to enlist a volunteer patient, apply healing-touch therapy and write up the results for the class. I hadn't planned on doing this assignment. However, events guided me differently.

During this time I was also participating in a discussion and prayer group held at a local Methodist church. I had been leading one of the prayer groups for several months when something unusual happened. One night two women attended who had not been there for a few weeks, and I had forgotten their names. I had to address them directly, so my lapse of memory might have been taken as a lack of interest. As I pondered what to do, one of the other members of the group looked at the women in question and said to one of them, "Susie, have you met Janet?" Susie responded, "Of course I know Janet." Then, as I thought gratefully of the divine guidance that had led this woman to bring their names to me, she turned to me and said, "Vernon, my arm hurts. Would you touch it and heal it?" I was amazed, because she knew nothing of my experience with healing-touch therapy or my interest in this area. I touched her arm and her pain was relieved. At that moment I knew I was to take the course in healing touch seriously and become an active student.

A friend who heard I was in the course volunteered to be my patient. A marathon runner in his late thirties, he had developed degenerative arthritis in his left ankle. He couldn't run, walked with a limp and had resting pain. Arthroscopic examination had revealed that the articular cartilage in the ankle had been eroded down to bone. When he walked, bone rubbed against bone. After our first healing-touch treatment, which lasted about five minutes, he was free of pain. Within two treatments he was walking without a limp, and within three weeks was running again. As of this writing, some nine years later, he is still running.

These and other experiences motivated me to leave the full-time practice of pathology in 1988 so that I could see clients as their physician and bring to them healing that was not available in the traditional approach to medical practice alone.

In the following pages, I will describe in more detail what I learned and how it can be applied to one's life.

Chapter 5

WHO WE ARE

While I was still in the full-time practice of pathology, I had sent for information about a special biopsy needle designed by Dr. Björn Nordenström, a Swedish radiologist. When I received the information I also received notice of a book he had written documenting his twelve years of research into the nature of the physical body as an energy phenomenon: *Biologically Closed Electrical Circuits: Clinical, Experimental and Theoretical Evidence for an Additional Circulatory System.*[70] I didn't order the needle, but I did order the book, and I was intrigued by what I found. Here was the documentation of biological/medical experiments confirming what I was learning from basic modern physics and spiritual teachings.

The body is associated with an energy field. This field exists within and around the body. What Dr. Nordenström had done was to demonstrate both in-vivo (in the body) and in-vitro (in the test tube) that this energy field is not produced by the body. The energy field produces the body. As quantum physics has demonstrated, all physical things are a manifestation of energy fields interacting in such a way as to produce the experience of substance. Dr. Nordenström demonstrated how this concept applies to the human body. From subatomic particles, to atoms, to molecules, to intracellular organelles, to cells, to tis-

sues and organs, to all the body's functions and anatomical relationships—all are manifestations of energy interaction.

Dr. Nordenström demonstrated that for there to be a chemical or
physical abnormality in the body there first has to be a disturbance in
the energy field that produces the body. He measured the energy field
of diseased tissue and compared it to the energy field of normal tissue.
Then he demonstrated that by changing the energy field electrically
and electromagnetically he could cause a reversal of abnormalities such
as the erasing of metastatic tumor nodules. Working with normal
breast tissue kept viable in the test tube, he could reorganize its structure by reorganizing its energy field.

In this and other pioneering work,[6] medical science is catching up
with quantum physics. Still, mainstream medicine, including most
medical research, is based predominantly on the Newtonian view and
has limited itself to the molecular, particulate world as a basis of
understanding disease—in spite of the fact that since the work of
Einstein[25, 76] and the law of relativity, we have known that Newtonian
physics is not a complete or accurate view of reality. The practical
application of this new information has introduced a new field that
some call energy medicine. As hypothesized in *Star Trek*, we may be
able to develop a technology that interacts directly with the body's
energy field, bypassing gross molecular therapies, to induce field
changes and body healing.

But there is yet a higher level of healing. Where does the energy
field of the body come from? The best evidence is that it has something to do with consciousness: thoughts and feelings that have an
effect on the energy field that makes the body. Indeed, it appears that
the energy that manifests the molecular and gross physical experience
of the body is itself a manifestation of consciousness or mind energy.
The energy field that makes the body is in the mind. There is now
plenty of scientific evidence to support these concepts. The differing

effects of fear and love on the energy field around the body can be seen in Kirlian photography.[117] Blair Justice, in a book entitled *Who Gets Sick*,[51] has reviewed the scientific literature researching the mind-body relationship. There is now evidence that if the mind is experiencing fear, DNA repair is impaired in the cells of the body.[34,51,53] DNA is the molecule that makes up our genes, which in turn are the macro-molecules that tell the cell what to do or not to do: whether to die or regenerate, or whether to regenerate abnormally, resulting in abnormal cell function or abnormal cell growth such as in cancer.

If the mind is anxious or depressed, there are corresponding demonstrable chemical changes in the brain. These neuro-chemicals (mood-chemicals) have been demonstrated to be produced in other parts of the body as well. It is important to realize that these chemicals are not the cause of our moods but the by-product. We can ingest external chemicals with a similar structure and experience a similar mood, but this is a synthetic mood. If the chemical is removed, our ordinary mood returns.

The effect of the mind on the body has also been demonstrated at the cellular level. Lymphocytes, the immune cells that protect us from infection, are negatively affected when experiencing fear. The deleterious effect of fear has been clearly documented at the organ level and organism level as well, as would be expected, since the organs and the body are made up of molecules and cells.[51]

Fear seems to be the primary culprit in disease, from simple infections to heart disease, stroke and cancer.

Fear is the emotional experience of stress. With fear there is always the associated feeling of guilt, although frequently it is not recognized. Fear results from the perception of threat, which is also associated with the perception of failure or potential failure. The feeling of failure is guilt. Guilt is usually disguised and projected as anger. All of this is also associated with the perception of loss or potential loss. The feeling of loss is grief: unresolved, this leads to depression. However it may be perceived, what is really grieved is the loss of Self.

Stress is not caused by the situation in which we find ourselves. It is the interpretation of the situation that induces the emotional experience. That interpretation is based on our perceptions—what we believe about ourselves and the world. Thoughts follow perceptions, and their emotional energy has "creative" power, out-picturing in the outer experience a reflection of the inner experience. What we perceive, to the extent that it represents our faith or belief system, becomes manifest. Evidence for these statements will follow.

Correction, then, is brought about through a change of perceptions, which is the purpose of our search and attempt to discover. What we have discovered is that we are not the body and are not made by the body. What we are is an energy field, an energy field of consciousness that is making the experience of a body. Energy fields are the domain of quantum physics.* In this domain, as proven by laboratory experiments, nothing is local or separate from anything else. Everything is connected to and has an effect on everything else, instantly, without limitations of time and distance. These statements reflect Bell's theorem of physics.

If the spin of an atom is altered experimentally in one location, it affects, in the same instant, the spin of another atom being observed at the same moment at some distance, no matter where it is located. In the case of identical but mirror-image photons traveling in opposite directions as a result of the effect of a mirrored prism on a beam of light, alteration in the polarization of one photon using a polarizing filter will affect the polarization of the twin photon, which is headed in the opposite direction some distance from the photon passing through the filter. In other words, particles in one location seem to

---

* References: 19, 38, 40, 52, 74, 75, 77, 115, 116, 122, 127, 128, 129, 130, 133.

know what is happening to particles some distance away.

In another experiment, subatomic particles in a linear accelerator approaching the speed of light were passed through a single-slit filter. Predictably, particles behaving as particles created a slit-like image on the detector at the end of the accelerator. Then particles were passed through a filter with two parallel slits. Instead of producing two parallel images, which would have been expected if the particles had behaved as particles, several parallel images were produced, none of which were exactly correspondent to the position of the slits in the filter. These experiments demonstrate the capacity of subatomic particles to behave as waves or as particles, depending on the method of observation.

In the double-slit experiment, the particles behaved like waves, which is not surprising since particles are made of energy and energy has wave-like characteristics. If you drop two stones adjacent to each other in a pond, the ripples from the two stones will intermingle. Those that are out of phase will cancel each other out. Those that are in phase will magnify each other. Those that are somewhere in-between with regard to phase will have a lesser effect than the two examples above. The two wave patterns combine as they come together, producing a third, new wave pattern. This is what happens in the double-slit experiments. The waves of energy passing between two slits behave like the ripples from the two stones in the pond, producing a new wave pattern. However, when the energy hits the detector at the end of the linear accelerator it behaves like a particle and produces an image of the new pattern—in this case, a multiple slit-like image.

But here is the most interesting part of the experiment. If only one particle is passed through the linear accelerator and the double-slit filter, it can only pass through one slit or the other. It would be expected then that as the particle hits the detector it would hit within the area that corresponds to one of the slits. In such an experiment, however, the particle fell into an area that corresponded to the interference wave pattern that would have resulted if the chamber had been flooded with particles passing through both slits at once. It seems that a single particle passing through one slit knows that there is another slit in the filter at another location and changes its behavior accordingly. The question in this case is: Who or what is doing the knowing? Could it be that unconscious aspects of the minds of the scientists conducting the experiments act as a non-local, omnipresent energy phenomenon, and are thus involved in the "knowing?" Could that unconscious "knowing" influence the results of the experiment?

Physicist Helmut Schmidt of the Mind Science Foundation in San Antonio devised some experiments to explore this question.* Dr. Schmidt used a radioactive source as a random-event generator (REG). The radioactive material in any short period of time would give off particle A or B, but there was no way to predict which, and it was just as likely to give off one as the other. Over a prolonged period an expected 50:50 distribution of particles would be released.

Dr. Schmidt had subjects concentrate on the REG with the intent to alter its randomness and to have either particle A or B released in preference to the other. The results were positive. The events were no longer random. The REG responded to the mind of the participant and preferentially released one particle over the other. His data has been scrutinized by other observers, including skeptics, and similar work has been done by other researchers. Schmidt demonstrated that consciousness is an active part of the pre-physical energy fields that determine subatomic events. Gross atomic events, such as the physical events in our lives, are manifestations of collections of subatomic events.

Dr. Schmidt showed that this impressive power of the mind can transcend time and even affect past events. In an extension of the

---

* References: 20, 99, 100, 101, 102.

experiment, the radioactive decay of the REG was recorded by the detector before the introduction of the conscious activity of the participant. After the decay had been recorded, the subject concentrated to bring about the desired results: the release of one particle in preference to the other. The results were again positive. The data showed that the experimenter could influence past events. However, if another person observed the findings of the detector prior to the experimenter's efforts to cause a consciously chosen result, he was less likely to be able to do so. Then it became a battle of minds. The first observation seemed to fix the event, but not inevitably, depending on the intensity of the focus of the minds involved.

These experiments show that in the realm of pre-physical energy the mind exists as an omnipresent, causal energy phenomenon that determines subatomic and then molecular events. In other words, the mind is very powerful.

Parapsychologists in some of our major universities are studying the telepathic ability of the mind to influence the thoughts and feelings of other minds some distance away.[1, 125] It has also been shown that minds can influence the energy of plants and the electromagnetic energy of metal. Psychokinesis, the movement of objects by the mind, has been well documented. In a visit to Moscow in 1990 I had the opportunity to view videos of research in psychokinesis. I believe they were valid recordings of events demonstrating the power of mind over matter.

Millions of people, including Western scientists and journalists, have observed Sai Baba, a holy man in India, materialize different types of objects, in addition to healing the sick.* I visited Sai Baba in India in 1989 and again in 1993 and saw him materialize ash and rings, coins, etc., in the palm of his hand, which was as close to me as this book is to you. There could have been no trickery involved. I

---

* References: 36, 41, 67, 68, 69, 97, 98.

brought two materialized objects back with me. And Sai Baba says, "The only difference between you and me is that I know who I am, and you do not yet know who you are." These phenomenal experiences of manifestation are not Sai Baba's greatest service, but they do demonstrate the potentially limitless nature of the mind of man when he is united with the truth of himself. However, Sai Baba's greatest gift to humanity is his love, including the teachings he shares and the benevolent activities he supports that affect the lives of so many.

These observations indicate that we are non-local energy fields of consciousness and that mind has the power to influence events beyond the reach of the body. If this were our perception, we would be able to release a lot of fear about lack of control and helplessness to affect the events in our lives in a positive way. Because the mind is omnipresent and powerful, our fears tend to become self-fulfilling prophecies and our lack of trust then seems justified. In the practice of medicine, making a physical diagnosis and establishing a prognosis based on past experience may become self-fulfilling, entrapping all concerned in a negative paradigm.

There is even more to be discovered. Where does the mind come from? Can we be sure of its wisdom and benevolence as an omnipresent powerful force? Up to this point everything I have discussed is based on scientific evidence. To proceed further we must go beyond science. We have the scientific precedents for taking such a step. Science has advanced as far as it has because of its willingness to go beyond itself. For example, before the work of Albert Einstein, all we had in the realm of science to understand physicality were Newtonian concepts, which are based on what the physical eye can see. To an extent these observations seem to work and can be expressed mathematically, but ultimately they are limiting.

Because he went beyond Newtonian physics, Einstein was perceived to have been tossing out long-held, valued beliefs. Probably because of his unorthodox views he was unable to obtain a university teaching position after receiving his advanced degree.[76] He got a job as a patent officer in Switzerland. There, working at a desk, without a laboratory or instruments, he came up with the law of relativity. What Einstein was describing could not be seen with physical eyes, not even through the physical instruments of that time. It was not until fourteen years after he first published his theory that the world developed the technology to prove that he was right. Those who observed Einstein work noted that he seemed to nap a lot. He would seem to awaken and continue his work. What he was doing was closing his eyes to the physical world and going within his mind, into the energy of consciousness, for a direct experience of wisdom from within—a mystical experience. The accuracy of his findings validates mysticism (inner knowing) as a source of wisdom.

To advance our understanding now, we must rely on mystical wisdom. This information is written in the ancient books of the world's religions, and is also available from more contemporary sources (see Appendix). According to this information there is a source mind, which is an omnipresent energy, the energy of consciousness, from which all energy and thus all things ultimately arise. This universal, omnipresent energy has all the attributes of mind. It knows. What it knows includes everything that can be known—omniscient. It thinks, and its thinking is the movement of energy into manifestation—omnipotent. It exists everywhere; there is nowhere that it is not—omnipresent. It also feels; that is, it has an emotional experience. What it feels is love. There is no alternative to love in its experience. It feels love because it is love. Love is energy and the energy state of the source mind. In our culture we call this source mind God.

The source mind (God) is self-aware, aware of knowing and feeling. Feeling love, it loves. It is the nature of love to love. In the experience of love's desire to love, the source mind extends itself by thinking. Its thinking is the movement of energy into manifestation so that it can love that which is manifest. Joy is inherent in the experience of love; thus as love is extended by thought, joy is increased.

This process is creation. Thus creation is motivated by love. What has been created? Everything that exists, including us. We are created by the source mind so that it can experience itself loving us. We are created to be loved.

Furthermore, according to both contemporary and ancient sources, we are created in God's image, meaning that we are energy of consciousness (mind), and we are also omniscient, omnipresent and omnipotent. We also are created self-aware, and as we pop into existence as a thought of God we pop into awareness of Self. We do not exist outside the mind of God, and the frequency of our mind energy is that of God, in His image. In this state we are aware of God, aware of omniscience and the experience of loving, of being loved and the joy of love. We also have the capacity to think. In our experience of love we desire to love. So we think for the purpose of loving. Our thoughts are the movement of energy into manifestation so that we can love that which is manifest. In so doing, we fulfill our function, for we are created to extend love and increase the joy of loving by co-creating in the energy of love, the energy frequency of God. We co-create with God as we think in love. As we love that which we create so too does God, just as God loves us. As the energy of all other created minds also exists in the mind of God, at the same energy frequency, so too do all other minds know and experience the joy of our creations just as we experience the knowing and joy of the creations of all other minds. Thus the experience of love is increased exponentially, as it is shared by all.

Each person can be thought of as the offspring of God, a son or daughter. According to the Christian Bible, Jesus knew this of himself. When he proclaimed that God was his Father, with whom he was one, the Pharisees accused him of blasphemy. His response was, "Is it not written in your Law, 'I have said you are gods'?" (John 10:34). He was referring to Psalm 82 in which the psalmist has God admonishing man for not acting like the sons of God that they are, but instead like mere men.

I have referred to our creation in the present tense. The implication of modern physics is that time is an illusion, a variable experience based on the position/perception of the observer. The experience of time is a manifestation of a pattern of thinking—in our case, collective thinking. This would confirm the mystical writings, from the ancient Vedas* to the contemporary *A Course in Miracles*, that clearly state that time is an illusion. Thus creation did not occur some time ago. Creation is occurring right now. Right now we are being created all wise and powerful, totally loving and completely joyous. That has not changed, and it never will. The difference between us and God is that, although we have the capacity to co-create, we did not create ourselves nor can we change how we are created. It is obvious that we can become unaware of all this, but we cannot change it. In other words, we can only change our awareness. In our earthly, human experience, we have become unaware of our wisdom, power, love and joy.

How did we become unaware and forget who we are? When we are created, we are given the freedom to chose our own thoughts. As we think a thought, our awareness will be in the energy of that thought. Our awareness is attached to the thoughts we have. We also experience the energy of thought as an emotion. A thought that is true has a characteristic energy frequency that is in harmony with the frequency of the energy of God, the source mind. The energy of truth is experienced as love and joy. As we think thoughts of wisdom (truth)

---

* The Vedas are ancient Sanskrit scriptures upon which Brahmanism (now called Hinduism) was based.[48,110,119] The faith of Abraham, the father of Judaism, had its origins in Brahmanism (AqG 10:1-15).[23] Of course, Christianity had its origins in Judaism. Muslims also trace their heritage back to Abraham.

to extend love and increase joy, our awareness is in the energy of those thoughts. We are free to think any thought in the energy of love and truth that we choose.

We are also free to think a thought that is not true. And we do. From the perspective of time, we may ask why we did that. The more appropriate question is, why are we continuing to do it now? Again, from the perspective of time, the process began before the experience of time—that is, beyond time. As one mind began to think a thought that was not true, a non-omniscient thought, other minds joined in, and it became a collective phenomenon involving many minds.

Certain predictable things happen when a mind begins to think an untruth. The awareness of the one holding the untrue thought will change and have different, lower energy characteristics (lower frequency). Thus the awareness of the mind as it thinks the untruth will begin to drop in frequency. It will then become unaware of the higher frequency energy of truth and the emotional experience of truth, which is love and joy, although this true nature of this now Higher Self remains unchanged. As the mind thinks the untruth it begins to experience emotionally the absence of love. That experience is what we call fear. As its awareness falls out of truth, it no longer knows wisdom. It no longer knows who it is, what its function is, its oneness with God, its purpose to love and be loved. It no longer experiences joy. It once knew but no longer knows. What was once known becomes only a perception which in time is like a memory. Because they are not direct energy experiences of knowing, perceptions and memories are subject to change and forgetfulness.

With awareness now in a state of untruth and fear, the mind perceives something is wrong. It thus experiences the feeling of failure, which, as mentioned earlier, is guilt. Fear is thus associated with the experience of guilt. Guilt intensifies fear, which leads to more guilt, which leads to more fear—and on and on. A self-perpetuating, increasingly negative energy dynamic is established in the mind.

Guilt is the worst experience a human can have. It is worse than the physical pain it ultimately causes. We would do anything to avoid it. This attempt to escape guilt leads to all the negative choices made in the world. In its negative awareness, the mind has a second mis-thought in an attempt to prove to itself and others that the first mis-thought was not wrong in the hope that the feelings of guilt will go away. The second mis-thought, however, being an untruth, intensifies fear, which leads to more guilt, which leads to more fear, and thus another negative, self-perpetuating, increasing energy dynamic is set up in the mind. The awareness drops lower in frequency. The mind then has a third mis-thought in an attempt to prove the second mis-thought is true, again hoping to escape guilt. But again it does not work, for the third mis-thought increases fear, which increases guilt, and on it goes as another negative energy dynamic is set up, placing a greater distance between awareness and the original energy of truth. Although the energy of truth is not experienced in awareness, the mind is not separate from it. A continual flow of higher energy is extended by the creator, is accepted by the higher aspect of the mind and reaches down to the fallen awareness even though the awareness, in its altered state, is unaware of its presence.

In its continued mis-thinking, the mind attempts to deny responsibility for its experience to avoid feeling guilty. Someone or something else is made guilty, and guilt is translated into anger. The threat is perceived apart from self, then blaming, complaining, and attack and defense begin, and feelings of separation increase. Concepts of levels of worth are devised in an attempt to justify blaming and complaining. In our own experience of lack of worth, we try to make someone less worthy so that we can feel more worthy and thus less guilty. The perception of scarcity develops out of the emotional experience of the lack of love and joy.

The mind in its mis-thinking attempts to replace what it lost with a substitute reality in which it attempts to define self as worthy and in which it tries to find a substitute source of joy. Substitutes, however, do not work, and because they are part of the system of mis-thoughts, more fear and guilt are generated.

In its negative state of awareness, the mind may choose to punish itself, hoping to appease the feelings of guilt by releasing them as pain and suffering. However, this doesn't work. The attack on self and its pain and suffering induce more fear and guilt.

Although the frequency of our awareness falls, our thoughts are still powerful. They still move energy into manifest but now at a lower frequency. Thus we make a lower frequency dimension and experience it as reality.

Never able to completely escape guilt by these means, the mind attempts to separate its awareness from these negative feelings. To some extent it is successful. This process of repression becomes an automatic, unconscious attempt to hide from our feelings. Thus we develop the subconscious mind. The mind at its lower level of awareness is not only unaware of truth, which is its real unchanged Self (higher consciousness); it is also unaware of many of its negative feelings and misperceptions. Consciousness has now become split into conscious and unconscious aspects with a further split within the unconscious between the higher nature (superconscious) and the lower (subconscious). This is actually a state of insanity. To be unaware of most of one's self is to be insane. The world can be thought of as a huge insane asylum, and we are all inmates, with the less insane attempting to help the more insane.

Although negative energy dynamics are repressed beyond our awareness, they still have the power to manifest. These repressed thoughts and feelings attract, cause and affect negative events around us, as well as make a negative experience of the body. These events seem to be beyond our control since we cannot, through the experience of the physical body, see the energy of our thoughts. We do not see the energy fields of physical manifestations or the energy of thoughts and feelings that are transferred and accepted or rejected among minds to produce a collective experience. By not seeing we attempt to preserve our innocence; but in so doing, we generate more fear from perceptions of helplessness and separation, leading to more mis-thoughts and mis-action, which in turn lead to more guilt and fear. And the cycle continues.

The physical world as we experience it today is a manifestation of aeons of collective mis-thinking by mankind. Since most of this miscreating is beyond our awareness, we assume that chance, the random forces of nature, or God is responsible. The paranoia of guilt causes many to assume that the negative events of life are the acts of an angry God punishing us. But God did not make the world this way; we did. We cannot blame nature either. The nature that we experience is a manifestation of the type of energy that we align ourselves with by the thoughts we choose to have. This emotional energy, most of which is in the subconscious, shapes the experience.

Our physical body is inherited from our mother and father. It is initially manifest through their energy. However, they did not make our minds. Our minds are created by God. There is substantial evidence from hypnotic regression studies and spontaneous memories that the mind predates the body.[56, 123] There is also ample corroborated evidence from studies of the near-death phenomenon that the mind continues to exist after death.* The mind is not made by the brain but uses and sustains the brain.

We actually have the capacity to focus our awareness anywhere in our omnipresent mind we choose. At birth we focus our mind energy into the physical body for the purpose of experiencing life through it.

---

* References: 2, 3, 5, 8, 37, 57, 65, 72, 92, 93, 94.

Light energy (photons) is reflected from the energy fields of the objects of our physical reality as we seem to look out into the world. This light passes through the pupil of the eye; the photons then stimulate the energy field of the retina onto which the energy field of our lens focuses them. This action stimulates the energy field of the optic nerve, which in turn stimulates the energy field of the visual cortex, creating there energy patterns that we learn to interpret as seeing. Thus it seems like we are inside our heads looking out.

This same general process applies to all the body's senses, creating the experience of being in the body while seeing, hearing and physically sensing a world that seems to be out there. But in fact, we are actually everywhere and "out there" exists in our mind. We have simply focused our attention into one energy aspect (image) of our omnipresent mind and have, quite literally, turned our awareness inside out—inside, looking out. What we experience through the energy field of our body seems to be an external, separate reality and is the only reality of which we are aware. This is an inherently frightening experience because it is not reality. The experience is associated with misperceptions of being separate, limited and vulnerable to the effects of something apart from us and out of our control.

We do not realize that out there is not outside the mind, and that the mind by thought determines what occurs out there, including the experience of the body. Although our body is initially made through the energy fields of our parents with their energy-genetic contributions, the incoming mind has the capacity to influence the body's molecular experience, including genetic combinations that occur at conception, and to influence and change genetic expressions after conception.

As children, what we learn about who we are comes through the physical experience of the body, but little of what we learn reflects reality. In this way we continue the effects of aeons of misperception as we perpetuate those perceptions either consciously or through the unconscious dynamics of repressed thought and emotional energy.

The process, however, begins even before birth. Prior to incarnating into the body, the individual focuses its awareness into the energy mileu of the family. At this point, the awareness of the individual is not limited to the physical brain. (It is also at this point that the incoming mind has the capacity to influence the genetic combinations of conception and fetal development.) In the state of expanded awareness, the individual telepathically knows what the father and mother-to-be, and other family members think and feel about the world and about the infant-to-be, which the individual begins to identify as itself. The incoming mind may absorb these energy patterns (the family's perceptions and feelings) as its own.

Immediately after incarnation and before the individual learns by trial and error how to use the physical brain, it still has expanded awareness. In other words, a newborn infant is aware at the "unconscious" level. That being the case, the infant is actually more conscious than its parents, although it cannot as yet use the new body to communicate that non-body consciousness. The infant continues to be influenced and programmed by the thoughts and feelings of its parents and others, all of whom reflect their culture. Those new belief systems are reinforced by what the child experiences through the body as he or she learns to use it to communicate with the physical world. At this point, although we are no longer consciously aware of the thoughts and feelings of those around us, we continue to be unconsciously impacted and influenced by them.

Many people believe in reincarnation. In this phenomenon, the individual may have experienced many lives and is born with the perceptions and emotional energy of previous life experiences. Those who do not believe in reincarnation will assume that this life is a first and only life experience. For our discussion, it doesn't matter which belief you accept. In my own experience, I have had occasion to work with people who carry with them memories and emotional scars from what seem to be previous life experiences.

What I have described in previous pages (the lowering of awareness through mis-thought and mis-deed) is the biblical "fall of man." This was a fall in consciousness. Incarnating into the physical world is like being born into sin. We are born into misperception and negative emotional energy, which we must learn to contend with. This is the biblical concept of "original sin."

The psychological dynamics of fallen man were analyzed by Freud,[16, 31] who coined the terms "super-ego" for the unconscious aspect, "ego" for the conscious aspect and "id" to refer to the body's appetites. Collectively these aspects are referred to by some as the ego system, or simply the ego. Carl Jung[29,49,50,71] and others recognized the collective nature of consciousness and a higher aspect of consciousness existing beyond the ego that can transcend ego limitations.

I have made some references to Judeo-Christian biblical concepts. Actually these concepts can be found in the teachings of all the world's major religions;[66, 68, 110] however, because most readers of this book will be from the Judeo-Christian background or will at least have been culturally influenced by it, I have chosen to make reference to that terminology. The purpose is not to promote Judeo-Christian traditions over others but to enhance communication and understanding.

The un-fallen higher aspect of self that remains at the same frequency of God corresponds to the Christ, or the Messiah. The extension of love from the highest dimension that followed man in his fall is referred to in Christian tradition as the Holy Spirit. The Holy Spirit is considered a distinct extension of God accepted in the Christ energy to heal the separation experience. It is an omnipresent energy of consciousness that knows both truth and the "realities" (illusion) of fallen consciousness. In its love and wisdom it contains solutions that honor the highest good of all. It brings love energy into lower frequency experience, resulting in the awareness of love and joy, and changes lower dimensional "reality" to reflect that love and joy. Although the frequency of love is stepped down to relate to lower frequency energy, it is in harmony with that of higher dimension. The love and joy thus experienced is not as great as that of higher dimension, but it is great enough to be experienced as total bliss while still in a lower dimensional body.

In Jewish tradition, this energy is referred to as Rauch Hakodesh, which literally means "Breath Holy." "Spirit" is from the Greek word meaning breath. Thus Holy Spirit literally means Holy Breath, referring to the ability to experience its effects without being able to physically see it. Jewish tradition also uses the word Sechinah, which refers to the feminine, nurturing aspect of God toward man; it also corresponds to the Holy Spirit. As held by the Christian tradition, Jesus through the energy of the Holy Spirit brought the Christ energy into the lower dimension of the earth. While he was in body, he maintained an open connection with higher dimension and was conscious of who he was as the Higher Self.

Great prophets and other enlightened ones have appeared in different cultures at different times, playing both an individually unique role and part of a collective role to awaken humankind to its fullest potential. Some appeared within the context of existing religious traditions, while from others new traditions sprang. Into their teachings the ego introduced errors of interpretation, yet in all of the world's great religions the truth can be found although the forms differ. As Paul taught, as recorded in 1 Corinthians 12:12-31, we are all one in the body of Christ—that is, the body of universal, unconditional love—the Higher Self that we all are.

How to evolve into that experience is discussed next.

Chapter 6

BEING WHO
WE ARE

Let's come back to the present. Here we are living a life containing fear and conflict, or it is at best less than totally happy. I have explained why we are lacking in joy and in a general way why we may be in physical or emotional pain. What can we do about it?

The problem is solved by the correction of the misperceptions that we have inherited and perpetuated, and allowing the negative emotional energy of those misperceptions to be changed. One basic misperception is that we are guilty. We are responsible for what we accept as truth and for how we behave based on what we choose to believe and think, but in fact we are not guilty. Based on the perceptions that we inherited at the time of incarnation and through life experiences, we have always done the best we could within the emotional energy that those perceptions generated. We are inherently good. We cannot be otherwise because we are created good.

The mind is like a sponge that has been dropped into a puddle of muddy water. Of course, the sponge absorbs the muddy water until it is soaked with it. When it can no longer tolerate the stench of the dirty water it searches and finds a way to squeeze it out and open up to receive clear water. In the process the sponge discovers it is still as pure as it has always been. The stench was from the dirty water. Furthermore, as the sponge cleans itself out it also cleans out the mud puddle.

As the mind is born into this plane, it absorbs the negative energy around it. We experience its pain; we act out from its fear and lack of wisdom and live with the results of our unhappy choices. When we experience enough pain we look for a different way, and in our willingness it is made available to us. In doing so, we heal the energy in our own mind and thus contribute to the healing of the planet by clearing out some of its negative energy. We then discover that our mind, like the sponge, is as pure as it always was. Rather than hang on to feelings of guilt for things we said and did, or did not say and do in the past, we should give ourselves the Purple Heart for coming here to experience the pain so we can heal it, and thus heal the world. In fact, that is precisely why we did come. We came to take on the planet and heal it as we heal our own experience of its pain. It was a given that we would absorb and experience the dirty water, that we would forget who we are and go through an awakening process.

The life we live, all of its events and relationships, are a reflection of ourselves. We must live it and have its experiences in order to learn what of ourselves we may want to change. In other words, our life experiences are like a self-portrait. If we were prevented from painting it, we would not have a picture of what needs to be changed, in order to express the masterpiece that reflects our true nature.

Another way to look at it is to see life as a long workshop in which we agree to participate in a psychodrama to bring up hidden emotions. In our negative relationships, we help each other bring up negative emotions so that they can be healed. When we feel insulted, someone is doing us a favor. We can see where we are vulnerable and where happiness is incomplete. Those we may have hurt also have a chance to see their weaknesses and discover their strengths. And in all of it, we are doing the best we can in total innocence.

Furthermore, all that happens individually and collectively because of the energy of mis-thinking is happening in the lower energy dimension of altered awareness, or altered consciousness, and as such is nothing more than fantasy manifest in fantasy. It is not held in the higher frequency of God; thus it is not eternal. In that sense, it is not real. When omnipotent minds fantasize, this is what happens—the world around us. It is experienced as reality, but it is no more real than the dream you had last night. The difference is that we keep returning to this dream, and it is a shared dream. It continues even now. You are dreaming that you are reading this book just as I dreamed I wrote it. If you commit a "sin" in a dream, when you wake up you are relieved when you realize that it never happened. So too it is in this dream of a physical world. Our goal, however, is to become conscious of the dream nature of the experience while we are in it so that we can become lucid dreamers, bring the dream to truth, and help each other awaken to it. Then we can choose to awaken to reality, which is beyond time, and beyond the ignorance and fear which cause us to be afraid of reality. In the process, it is helpful to remind ourselves and others that we are dreaming so that we do not resist awakening and slip back into an unpleasant dream of fear.

In addition to the intellectual work of correcting perceptions, there are other things the mind can do to facilitate healing. Fear does not heal itself. It is self-perpetuating. Only love, the higher and more powerful form of energy, can heal fear. When love interfaces with fear, the lower frequency energy begins to change. When the low frequency of fear and its translations—anger, guilt and grief—are changed back to the higher frequency of love, fear no longer exists. There is only love.

How do we access love to heal fear? The opening for the influx of love to occur is willingness. Our will is expressed by the thought we choose to hold. Everything occurs through thought. We make the world around us by thought. We activate our connection with everything around us by thought. When we think about something or someone, there is an energy exchange. We can influence or be influenced depending on our intent and the degree of vulnerability caused by our misperceptions and lack of vigilance. We are almost constantly thinking about people, things and events in the world we see. Because there is so much fear in this world, we absorb it and experience its thoughts.

Fortunately our minds are omnipresent not only in this third-dimensional space-time experience. We are omnipresent throughout all dimensions, including the highest dimension, the dimension of pure love—God. We can activate our connection with this dimension and access its higher energy by thought. We think in words and symbols. Thus we may think about being one with God to experience the love of God, or we may visualize symbols such as light to represent love and imagine it surrounding us and affecting our experience. If you are uncomfortable with the word God or your belief does not encompass the use of that word, it is enough simply to think of something good beyond your awareness for good, and the connection will be activated. You may also think about being one with the highest aspect of your self. Or you may use a name that represents a connection to God, such as the name of a prophet, saint or some member of the hierarchy of a particular religion. If we feel personally or more emotionally connected to a religious personality who has demonstrated God's love, the use of that person may make the connection stronger for us. It matters not to God or to love what we call it. It is our intent, or will, expressed in thought that activates the connection.

In our culture, the process I have been describing is called prayer. I will use that word since it is shorter than saying "activate our connection with the higher energy by thought." As we pray with willingness to be free of the energy of fear and its translations, we access the higher energy that raises the vibrations of the lower frequency energy. This results in a growing awareness of peace, love, joy, gratitude, compassion, affection and trust. This love is an extension of energy from the highest level of consciousness down to lower dimensional experience.

As I have said, the omniscience of this energy of higher consciousness knows both truth and misperception. Its wisdom contains the solution to any problem and honors the highest good of everyone. This energy offers a new way of interpreting our experience and a new understanding of what the experience does or does not mean. With the willingness to release fear there must also be a willingness to release the perceptions that generate fear or its translations. If we want to experience love and the peace and joy of love, we must be willing to accept its wisdom. This may come into our awareness intuitively or through information brought to us by the synchronicities of life. Would we rather be right or happy? (ACIM T-29.VII.9)[17] If we think that happiness lies in being right, which is what our culture seems to teach, we are in for disappointments that may ultimately lead to a willingness to accept another answer.

As this higher energy begins to affect our minds, even before it completely affects our conscious awareness, it reaches out through our omnipresent energy field and begins to change the world around us to reflect love and wisdom back to us. The world then becomes a place in which it is easier to remain happy. This change includes the energy and molecular experience of the body; thus physical healing occurs. It also influences the people around us, calling forth from them their best responses to us to the extent that they are willing. If they are unwilling to reflect love, they will leave us alone because their energy field will be incompatible with the higher energies coming through us. Our relationships will improve. Our circumstances will improve. We will become more prosperous. This kind of energy will influence the animals and plants around us. Our pets and livestock will be calmer and our plants will grow better. It will even affect the quality of our experience with the inanimate things around us. For instance, our appliances will work better. It is not that our happiness depends on these changes, for because of our direct experience of inner joy, we are less perturbed by events around us.

Prayer made the difference in my own experience of illness, broken relationships, financial problems and depression. My emotional experience became one of great peace and love. Certain people and situations no longer annoyed me. For example, I used to be annoyed in traffic when I found myself behind a slow driver, often someone elderly who was probably in no condition to drive faster. Now, instead of being annoyed, I experience overwhelming love for the driver and focus that love on him. Heavy traffic still exists, but my reaction to it is different, and it seems to have no effect on my life or schedule.

I discovered, or I should say it was shown to me, that a minimum dose of prayer is necessary to maintain a higher state of consciousness and a charmed life experience. In my own experience of healing I reveled in the freedom from pain and the new experience of the joy of love. Then life offered me new opportunities in the form of new challenges, which brought out residual fears. The peace slipped away and the temptation to be irritated became more and more difficult to resolve. I wondered about this phenomenon, and as I had learned to do, I prayed for a solution. The answer came in the form of dreams and meditative visions. The message was that I needed to activate more my connection with the higher spiritual energies. One aspect of the solution was to pray aloud three times daily, for approximately five minutes. Heretofore my practice had been one daily formal prayer period that was not necessarily verbal.

The results were almost immediate. I spontaneously felt overwhelming love toward people whom I had previously been tempted to judge with irritation. That irritation had been compounded by a sense of guilt, because I judged myself for having the feelings. The problem was solved by my continued willingness to love and the simple practice of verbal prayer three times daily to focus on that intent.

Why pray out loud? It is not that God needs us to do so, but we may need to. If we verbalize a thought, we are more focused on that thought and thus put more energy into it, opening ourselves to receive more. In like manner, if we ritualize a prayer with some physical activity, we are putting even more of our energy into it and thus reap even greater benefits. This is the value of religious ritual. We, of course, can put just as much energy into a silent prayer, but in verbal or ritualized prayer we will generally be more consistent in doing so.

The formula I suggest for these formal prayer periods is to begin with gratitude. Gratitude is like the key that opens the door. It is a component of love, and as we focus on gratitude we align ourselves with the higher energies. First, in an abstract way, begin by verbalizing gratitude for the love of God, your creation in it, and the blessings it brings to you. Then, more specifically, acknowledge gratitude for the good things you have experienced, no matter how insignificant, no matter how much you may have taken them for granted. Verbalize this as if in a conversation.

Then verbalize the need and desire for healing. The need is always for the release of fear or its translations (anger, guilt or sadness), and the release of the perceptions that generate those feelings. This process always involves some form of forgiveness—a release of judgment of self and others with a willingness to experience love and joy. We need not attempt to generate these feelings, for we cannot. We need only focus on our willingness to experience them and have them operate in our lives. The feelings already exist. We simply open ourselves to receive them, and in so doing release and surrender the old feelings and perceptions. After acknowledging the need, we verbalize release and surrender.

The next step is commitment. Release commitments to old perceptions and desires and commit to the experience of the love of God directly from within, independent of the world around us. Commit to love and the peace it offers, without first requiring some change in the world. Thus we let go of the need to fix someone else or solve a problem so that we might be happy, but instead open up to happiness now. If we commit to love and joy now, its energy will operate through our unconscious energy field and begin to generate solutions and, if appropriate, give us the ideas and the actions to take to accept the solutions. As the Bible says, "But rather seek ye the kingdom of God, and all these things shall be added unto you" (Luke 12:31). To repeat: we must let go of the attachment to outcome in the material plane. If we do, we will become open to higher energies, which will be free to bring about the perfect outcome. As our highest good is honored, so too is the highest good of everyone else. Others are not separate from us, and their highest good is not divergent from ours. At the outer-mind level, we are not likely to know the best solution. We must be willing to trust the wisdom of love, and to commit to it.

The next step in the prayer formula is acceptance. Verbalize the acceptance of the love of God as peace, joy and the capacity to experience love and compassion toward all, without exception. Then verbalize the acceptance of love as the problem solved, the situation healed. Accept love as a healed body, a healed relationship, better finances, a better work situation or whatever outcome is appropriate. The real problem, of course, is the fear and negative perception that allowed or attracted the situation or blocked change. Verbalizing acceptance will help to uncover and release subconscious fears and blocks. Yet even as we accept a vision of the problem solved, we must also remain flexible and unattached to a specific outcome, knowing that whatever the outcome is it will be perfect and there will be nothing to fear. There will be only love in it. It is important to remember that the secret to success is willingness to be peaceful and happy now, before specific changes occur. Then changes will occur easily and spontaneously and will align the events of our lives with our highest good. Visualizing the problem as solved may help to align thoughts with the peace needed to solve it. The outcome may be different than our initial vision, because of our inability to reach a higher understanding at that point. However, the emotional content of the outcome will more than match the emotional experience of what we were able to envision.

Following this acceptance mode, I recommend a period of celebration with gratitude for the peace and joy of love and the resolution of problems.

The Formula for Prayer

Gratitude	Express gratitude for love and its manifestations.
Release	Surrender all fears, anger, guilt, sadness and the false perceptions upon which they are based.
Commitment	All the things you want in the world is how much you want to experience this love from God.
Acceptance	Accept the out-picturing of God's love in all aspects of life: health, happiness, success, prosperity and good relationships.
Celebration	Once again acknowledge gratitude.

The duration of the prayer period does not have to be exactly five minutes, but it should preferably be at least several minutes. I must hasten to add, however, that no prayer, long or short, silent or verbal, is wasted. There is much advice available on how to pray and what form to use. Listen to the advice of others and then come up with the form of prayer that is most comfortable for you now. That will be the right one.

In addition to formal periods of prayer, frequent silent prayer is important. Any time we are upset, a quick silent prayer for release and for another way to see the situation is in order.

Prayer as I have described it may be thought of as the active opening of our connection with the energy of higher dimension for healing. There is also the important, more passive experience of receiving. We may think of prayer as talking with God for a specific or general purpose, or simply for the experience of communion in love and gratitude. The latter is the highest form of prayer. We also need to listen, to allow the mind to be quiet so that it can receive. This may not involve the reception of specific information, although it may be experienced that way, but it does allow a higher energy to flow into our energy field in this lower plane of experience. Psalm 46:10 of the Bible states, "Be still and know that I am God." The Psalm refers to a physical battle, which serves as a metaphor for the struggle in our minds caused by thoughts of fear and conflict. If we were simply to stop thinking for a while, we would realize what is meant by the affirmation from *A Course in Miracles*, "I need do nothing" (ACIM T-18.VII). [17] We would find that after a short period of non-thinking we would become very peaceful, and with a somewhat longer period that peace would evolve into bliss. Then we would experience what is meant when it is said that we are already joyous.

The mind can be likened to a lake with a muddy bottom. As the currents flow, the mud is stirred up. When the sun shines on the lake it does not penetrate below the surface. If the currents were to stop, the mud would settle out and light would penetrate the surface and reach the bottom. There it would stimulate the seeds of water plants, which would grow over the bottom of the lake and absorb the mud. Then, when the currents flowed again, there would be no mud to stir up; the clear water would sparkle in the sunlight, and the lake would remain clear, beautiful and healthy. The mud in the bottom of the lake represents the fear caused by our misperceiving; the currents are our thoughts, which reflect our misperceptions and stir up the fear. When we stop thinking, the fears that accompanied the negative thoughts no longer block the higher energies. The light penetrates the mind and awakens ancient memories of truth. The foliage that covers the bottom of the lake and absorbs the mud represents the new perceptions that reflect truth growing from seeds of wisdom. No fear is generated by these perceptions or by the thoughts that accompany them.

The mind was created to create, and we create by thinking. Thus it is not in our nature not to think. Although we can learn to discipline our minds to achieve that non-thinking state, simply by concentrating on a thought or thoughts that do not distract us from truth we can reach and remain in a state of peace. When the thought is in harmony with the energy of truth, the peace of God then flows into our awareness and into the world that our thoughts make. It does not matter what the thought is as long as it allows us to be peaceful and is compatible with love. In my case, I imagined that I was out in my sailboat because sailing brought me great peace. So I focused on a very complex thought that involved an entire scene: the boat, its sails, and the waves and spray. I went sailing in my imagination. When thoughts of the past or future entered my mind, I gently sent them away by refocusing on the sailing scene. After I developed more discipline, I used less complex thoughts, such as the affirmation, "I am the peace of God." Or I stared at a candle flame and became totally absorbed in the visual experience; or listened to peaceful music and became totally absorbed in the auditory experience. I also counted my breath over and over again, one through twelve, and became focused on my breathing. The goal was to become totally involved in the physical activity of breathing in order to let go of thoughts that were beyond the experience of the moment.

Physical activity such as running or other forms of exercise may be used as the focal point of concentration. This more active form of focusing the mind away from troubling thoughts is very useful when the mud is especially thick and it seems difficult to stop the flow of negative currents. Chanting the positive thought out-loud may be used in these situations as a way of keeping the mind focused.

In our culture, this process of stilling the mind for the experience of inner peace is usually called meditation. My recommendation is to meditate twice daily, immediately after awakening in the morning and again in the evening. Establish the intent of the meditation with a prayer. Meditate for 15-30 minutes each session. The beginner should begin with shorter periods so that the frustration of not initially being able to discipline the mind does not build up too much negative energy. With practice, it will become natural, and you will ultimately develop the ability to instantly go into a meditative state.

With continued meditation, in addition to experiencing peace and then bliss, you will usually begin to have visual experiences. The most common is the experience of beautiful waves of colors folding in and out in the darkness behind the closed eyelids. You may use the colors as a focal point of concentration to maintain the thought-free state. In this experience, you are actually seeing the higher spiritual energies. You may also experience a body rhythm, such as a gentle swaying or subtle (or not-so-subtle) vibration. Again, this experience may be used as the focal point of concentration. The goal of the meditation is to experience peace, and that is sufficient. However, one may also have useful and enlightening visionary experiences or the reception of information in what I call "stereophonic knowing." There may also be the experience of hearing a voice with peaceful, gentle instruction.

In the early stages of entering meditation, you may experience energy or information from the collective subconscious (negative consciousness). This will be a harmless experience. Simply by re-focusing on the truth—that there is nothing to fear—you will quickly pass through it. When information comes, ask what its source is and you will be shown whether it is from higher consciousness or lower consciousness. As your consciousness opens up to and invites in more love, you will become less susceptible to these lower energies. If you always set the intent of the meditation with a prayer, your connection with a higher source will be insured.

After you have meditated regularly for a while, you will notice some changes in your life experience. The energy that is expressed through you will become positive and strong. In the past you may have had the experience of walking into a building or into a room full of people and feeling uneasy, sad or irritable. You probably absorbed the dominant energy in the room. After meditating regularly for a number of months, rather than being negatively influenced by the negative feelings of the people around you, they will take on your more positive energy and begin to feel better. Arguments will be resolved; people will become positive; and wise solutions to problems will be found in the group process. Free will, however, operates. If someone does not want to become peaceful, he doesn't have to, but he will not be able to stay in your energy field, which is more powerful, and remain negative. The experience will be uncomfortable for him, and he will find some excuse or unconsciously devise a reason to leave. Then you won't have to deal with him. However, if you judge the person for leaving, or judge his leaving as being a threat to you, you will have allowed your own energy to drop back into fear. Then he may return with less than optimal results.

With regular meditation, you will also find that you will become smarter, more spontaneously humorous, happier, healthier and more prosperous in all aspects of your life. The energy of your Higher Self will be expressed through your personality and into your experience in the physical world. All this can be achieved by simply spending time every day doing nothing. Remember, twice daily for 15-30 minutes. If you don't get the full time in, don't be discouraged. Any amount of time is of benefit. The energy you seek loves unconditionally; thus to receive the most benefit, you must be willing to be all-inclusively, unconditionally loving and happy right now.

In addition to prayer and meditation, another important activity falls into the category of vigilance. Every thought we have has an effect. There is no such thing as an idle thought. Our emotional experience and the events of our lives will be determined by the quality of our thoughts. We may not see the connection between our thoughts and these events, for there may not be an instantaneous reaction in the linear experience of time. We cannot see the energy of thought; nonetheless, it is useful to begin to think of thoughts as being as real as actions. As we have discussed, thoughts that reflect truth will be associated with the emotional energy of love, which we will also experience as peace and joy. Thoughts that do not reflect truth will be associated with some form of fear, which we may experience as guilt, anger or sadness. The emotional energy of our thoughts is their creative power, and it creates that which reflects itself. Anger and guilt create angry and punishing experiences. Fear and sadness create frightening and sad experiences. Therefore, we must become vigilant about every thought. We must witness the thought and analyze it. Is it loving? What kind of feeling do we have with it? If the thought is negative, send it away and choose a positive one. As we think thoughts that reflect truth, we bring peaceful energy into our minds. We may not initially be conscious of the peace because of the amount of subconscious fear from all the old negative perceptions and thinking. With each positive thought, we heal the negative energies in our subconscious and reprogram it to a new pattern of thinking, until positive thinking and a continual awareness of peace become spontaneous.

It may be a new idea to think that we can actually choose our own thoughts and even stranger that we can choose how we feel, because we are so accustomed to reacting passively to the world around us with old patterns of thinking. When negative thoughts just pop into our minds, we allow ourselves to be sucked into a vortex of negative thought energy until such time as we realize that we have a choice. These negative thoughts may come to us from our subconscious, or from the collective subconscious.

If someone around us is into negative thinking, those negative thoughts might pop into our own awareness. We may have no idea where a thought comes from; and even though it may not be from our own subconconscious, if we accept it, it becomes ours and begins to affect us and our experience. We may have been taught as children not to drink out of other people's glasses to avoid catching their germs; better that we take care not to think their negative thoughts, for in thinking them we become vulnerable to negative energy. Dr. Elizabeth Kubler-Ross[54] said in one of her talks that if we have a thought and hang on to it for more than fifteen seconds, it is ours. If we expel the thought before then, it won't affect our energy. A thought, however, can be healed and its effects transformed at whatever point we become aware of it and choose to change.

Some examples of thoughts that reflect the truth are: I am totally innocent, and so is everyone else; everyone is equal; there is no one more or less than I; everyone is totally worthy, so worthy that their value is beyond evaluation; I cannot be offended, insulted or attacked; there is no scarcity, loss or lack.

It is true that we may experience attack, scarcity, loss or lack, and in a variety of ways, but this occurs only if we persist with the negative thinking that is compatible with such experiences. We may be vulnerable to becoming involved in negative events directed our way from others because of our lack of vigilance, even though we are not initially thinking about the specific event. We may in the moment accept a negative thought and perception projected onto us from another, or we may more actively manifest/attract them from our own repressed negative emotions. As these events emerge, they can be transformed immediately and the negative emotions healed as we refocus with positive thinking.

A fourth activity or tool for healing is what I call focus, which is similar to vigilance. Love is the energy that we want. It is the most powerful energy and is totally benevolent and wise. Love loves. So simply focus on loving everyone and everything without exception. The mind cannot be compartmentalized. If we are angry at a person, institution or thing, that anger permeates all the images in our mind, as well as our own body and its experiences. Anger is like a machine gun that shoots 360 degrees out of both ends of the barrel. The one who pulls the trigger gets most of the bullets. Anger comes back to its source as guilt. Another way to look at it is that the unconscious perceives no separation. Anger at another is interpreted as anger at self. In like manner, anger at self is experienced as anger toward others.

How do we focus on love? Simply by choosing to think a loving thought, such as, "I love you." To everyone you see no matter how casual the encounter, make the silent affirmation, "I love you." Do an inventory of the past and affirm love for everyone remembered. Exclude no one. Anytime you think of a future encounter with someone, focus on your love for him or her and see that person as being loving. Trust is a component of love. You must reach for what you lack. If you think someone is going to cheat you or cause harm in any way, choose to think this thought in reference to that person: "I trust my brother with whom I am one." You are not stating a falsehood, for there is within that person that which is totally trustworthy. Love is the most powerful energy, and when you focus on it during an interaction with another, the other person must allow his own fear to be healed and become trustworthy as his own love comes forth; or he will have to get out of your energy field and leave you alone, as his own energy field is incompatible with your higher, stronger energy. He will then not be able to cause you harm. He may go away complaining, but words can cause you no harm unless you believe them. Others will come in and fill the void and more than satisfy the needs of the situation. Then two people choosing to experience love will increase the experience for both.

As I have said, in our culture it has been my experience that eighty per cent of the people will accept love when it is offered. It doesn't matter how dire the situation is. As we recognize the need for healing and focus on love and trust, the situation will be transformed. Someone may come up behind you on a dark street at night and put a knife to your throat or a gun in your back; if you are willing to love and focus on trust, you will walk away unscathed. You will not read about such encounters in the newspapers, for the media usually only report on cases of victimization, but I am personally aware of several such cases and have had my own less challenging experiences, so I know it works.

Because of repressed negative emotions and perceptions in the subconscious, it is best to consciously choose to focus on love and trust, ever vigilant for the loving thought, taking no situation, encounter, or experience for granted. Otherwise a negative experience may begin to manifest when we least expect it and seem to get the upper hand in a moment of surprise as we slip into forgetfulness. In those "for granted" lapses our awareness may wander into "idle" thinking which has nothing to do with the experience at hand but may be subtly negative, and thus not incompatible with a negative experience. Yet, as mentioned earlier, at any point that we remember and focus on love, a negative situation can be transcended. Of course, at that point of remembering, we also realize the situation is not truly negtive, but is an opportunity to extend love and heal unhappy emotions. As the subconscious is healed, this vigilance will take less conscious effort. Our thoughts will become spontaneously more positive.

In truth there is nothing to fear, absolutely nothing. You may release all fears now and have a peaceful journey through life, enjoying the excitement of remaking the world with love and expressing love through your creative experiences. Your life will be beautiful and bring joy to many. It will not be boring. We do not have to be scared to death to know we are alive. We do not have to experience grief to know what happiness is like. Bliss does not need an opposite for us to be aware of its presence. Happiness is an inherent experience of our true nature.

Gratitude is also a component of love. Focus on it. If someone seems repulsive, use this affirmation: "God, I am grateful for the presence of this person so that I may learn of my love for him." If the situation looks terrible, look for and ask for something to be grateful for. Remember, your emotional energy will manifest like itself. If we remain in the energy of ingratitude, that energy will create a situation in which it is difficult to feel grateful. Reach for a feeling of gratitude first; then the situation will begin to change and will evolve as a reflection of the energy of gratitude. Then it will become easier to feel grateful.

One of my clients was having great difficulty in feeling gratitude for the presence of his supervisor. However, he was a good student and practiced the lessons he was learning. Three weeks later, at his next appointment, he had startling news. His supervisor had been unexpectedly transferred! We can correctly assume that the transfer was also for the supervisor's highest good.

Respect is also a component of love. Reach for respect for another, for all that is part of him. Respect his beliefs even if you disagree with them. This does not mean that we shouldn't express our views when, while feeling peaceful, it seems appropriate to do so. Continue to focus on respecting the other person and his beliefs while sharing your views. He will unconsciously pick up your feeling of respect, which is what he really wants. He may have thought that if he were right and his views held sway, he would get the respect he missed. But once he feels from you the respect he wants, he will become less fearful and will no longer need to be right. Then compromise will occur, and his mind will open to the possibility of change.

Vigilance and focus are essentially the same activity, and both are essentially the same as prayer. We align ourselves with truth through thought. Thus, every thought becomes a prayer. Prayer may be supplicative or affirmative. If we affirm the truth with every thought, we are in affirmative prayer and are thus following the instructions of St. Paul when he said in his letter to the Thessalonians, "Pray without ceasing." The whole instruction may be found in I Thessalonians 5:16-18: "Be forever joyous. Pray without ceasing. Give thanks in every circumstance." Few people can accept this as a practical instruction. But it is, and it can be accomplished. Ultimately it is essential for us to master it; and we will do so. The choice we have is when.

If we are awake sixteen hours of the day, we will have approximately 19,200 thoughts, assuming that each component of a series of thoughts lasts about three seconds. Each thought has an effect. Some are positive but many are negative; thus we create beauty and chaos side by side. Some aspects of our lives are good, but we also have some unpleasant experiences. Our lives are like a mixed dream, in part pleasant and in part nightmarish. The goal is to transform our lives until they are totally pleasant. This goal is not only possible, it is our birthright. There is nothing unloving about wanting total happiness. The world needs it.

Since there are so many negative thoughts barging into our minds from past negative energy dynamics maintained in our own subconscious and from the collective subconscious, it may be useful to have a list of positive thoughts or affirmations on hand to recite over and over again to keep our minds out of trouble. *A Course in Miracles*[17] and the "I AM" Discourses[33] are excellent sources for healing affirmations.

You might be wondering, "If my mind is so powerful why haven't my worst fears come to pass?" The answer is that we are never free of love. No matter how great our fears are, they are seldom realized to their fullest. Even if a negative experience goes as far as death, we will then have the realization that, in fact, one cannot be killed. We are not bodies. The mind does not die, and it will torture itself only so much before it seeks another way.

The Formula for Healing

Prayer	Pray three times daily, aloud, for approximately five minutes; silently, as needed.
Meditation	Meditate twice daily for 15-30 minutes.
Vigilance	Monitor each thought, choose to think only positive thoughts.
Focus	Focus on love, trust, gratitude and respect for everyone and everything in every situation.

It is not enough to be encouraged by these ideas, although that is a good first step. One must eventually, in some form or another, do the things I have suggested. It seems difficult but does not have to be. This formula is certainly better than a lifetime of suffering or, at best, quiet desperation. If you went to see a doctor because of an illness and he gave you a bottle of pills, you would take them if you thought they would make you well. This formula is my prescription to you. You do not have to believe that it will work; just accept that it might and do it. You will experience only positive results with no unpleasant side-effects.

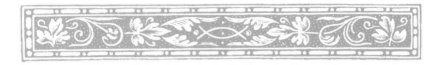

Chapter 7
MORE ON PRAYER
(AND THE ROLE OF FORGIVENESS)

As we activate our connection to higher energy through thought, we can also activate that connection for others. Many people are unaware of this inner potential and do not know how to access it. We can do it for them. Free will still operates, but as I have said, most people will accept the energy of love and allow their fear and its side-effects to be healed. Love will seek out their highest good. We will not be infringing on their rights, because the choice to accept love now or reject it is up to them.

This process is called intercessory prayer. The best thing we can do for others is to pray for them. In doing so we are harnessing the most powerful and benevolent force in the universe. Even if they are unable to accept love now, it will be there for them when they are ready. No prayer is wasted and every prayer has an effect, although it may not be immediately experienced.

My sources of information about intercessory prayer are mystical teachings, my own personal experience and the experience of others. There is also scientific validation of the effectiveness of intercessory prayer. Dr. Randy Byrd, a cardiologist, reported in the *Southern*

Medical Journal, 1985,[9, 51] on his double-blind study done in the coronary unit of San Francisco General Hospital. In the study, 393 coronary-care patients were randomized into two groups. One group was prayed for; their names were assigned to prayer groups. The other group of patients was not assigned to a prayer group. Neither the patients nor the hospital staff knew which patients were in which group. After a ten-month period the results were analyzed, and even the skeptical were amazed. There were significantly fewer complications in the prayed-for group as compared to the control group. Only three patients in the prayed-for group required antibiotics compared to sixteen in the control group. Six patients in the prayed-for group experienced pulmonary edema as opposed to eighteen in the control group. None of the patients in the prayed-for group required intubation while twelve patients in the control group did.

If a drug had been responsible for this kind of improvement, millions of dollars would have been spent on its development and marketing. Yet hospitals have not, as a routine, set up prayer groups for their patients. Admittedly, more study would be useful to convince the world of the efficacy of prayer. But since the procedure has no side-effects and minimal cost, why wait?

More scientific documentation of the power of prayer can be found in Dr. Larry Dossey's book, *Healing Words*.[20]

Since we learn better from shared experience than from relating abstract concepts, I will share some of my own experiences with intercessory prayer. Several years ago my youngest daughter, who was fourteen at the time, came down with infectious mononucleosis. One evening, after she had been sick for about a week, I sat on the side of her bed to comfort her. She had a high fever and her throat was covered with exudate and was very painful. She was also suffering from generalized aching and pain. It was early in my own spiritual journey or I wouldn't have waited so long to do what I did next. I had just placed my hand on her hot, feverish forehead, when—out of my strong desire to help her—came the inspiration to pray. I let my hand drop away from her forehead and prayed silently, with great intensity. After a few moments, I placed my hand back on her forehead and to my amazement it was completely cool. Her fever was gone. Within a few days she was completely well.

In another incident, I had flown to Texas to visit my mother, who was in a coma, apparently approaching death. I had to fly home that night because of other obligations. My medical judgment was that she would be dead within twenty-four to forty-eight hours. But I did not pronounce this judgment. Instead I waited until I had the opportunity to be alone with her, at which time I prayed aloud for her healing. When I prayed, I did not fixate on any certain outcome. I expected that she would die. Yet I was not totally surprised when my brother called the next morning to tell me something unexpected had happened: our mother had awakened that morning bright and alert. I did not see her alive again, however, for a month later she went to sleep and did not wake up. As my brother later said, she seemed to have surveyed her situation and made a conscious choice to leave.

While I was at lunch one day with a neurosurgeon, he related to me the following unusual case. He had operated on a woman with a tumor deep in the mid-brain. A three-centimeter lesion had been demonstrated by CAT scan (computer assisted tomography), which is a very refined X-ray procedure giving precise imaging of internal structures. Because of the tumor's location, it was considered inoperable. However, the surgeon planned a biopsy to obtain tissue in order to determine the tumor type to see if chemotherapy or X-ray therapy would be helpful. This procedure was done six days following the last CAT scan. A probe was placed through a burr hole cut in the woman's skull and a specimen was taken, using X-ray guidance. Frozen section was done immediately on the tissue. The pathology report came back:

"normal brain tissue." He made another burr hole, took a second specimen and again the report came back normal tissue. He tried a third
time and got the same report. In frustration he gave up. Two days later
he repeated the CAT scan and found no tumor. I asked him what the
family thought about this. He responded, "Thank God they believe
in miracles."

Because I was at the time investigating miracles, I decided to
review the case. I viewed the films, which were subsequently present-
ed in radiology and neurosurgical conferences; there is no doubt of the
existence of the lesion. I also reviewed the patient's hospital record,
and then sought family members to interview. The patient had experienced progressive central-nervous-system symptoms beginning
approximately three months before the tumor was discovered. These
symptoms had been preceded by significant family stress.

The patient and her family were very religious, and they engaged
in much prayer activity after the diagnosis of the tumor. The night
before surgery the family priest went to the patient's bedside for a lay-
ing-on of hands healing prayer service. This was the only thing I could
find that was somewhat out of the ordinary. The family, in any event,
is convinced that their prayers resulted in a miraculous healing, and the
circumstantial evidence strongly suggests such a conclusion.

Of course, intercessory prayer is not limited just to physical problems. Any condition or situation can be positively affected. One father
was greatly concerned about his son, who as a young man had become
caught up in the drug world. As a user the son's life had begun to fall
apart, so the father began to pray with great intensity. Following the
initiation of this effort, someone informed on the son. His apartment
was raided and drug-weighing devices were found. He was charged
with possession with the intent to sell and was brought before a judge
who was notorious for putting first-time offenders away for at least
two years. The son was convicted, but to the amazement of everyone

the judge demonstrated unusual leniency, sentencing him to six months in the city jail with a work pass. The pass meant he could solve some of his financial problems, and the six months in jail were just what he needed to get him off drugs. At first it was thought that the arrest of this young man was a tragedy, but it turned out to be a blessing. This incident shows that it is important in doing prayer work to let go of attachment to outcome.

All prayer is intercessory, for we do not live in isolation. Many other people are involved in our lives, so when we pray for ourselves it affects all who share in our experience. When my wife was working as an operating-room nurse, a young woman insisted that she be given the opportunity to pray aloud prior to anesthesia. Her surgery was the one operation that day that went without a single flaw: no missing instruments, no lost sponges, none of the minor or major inconveniences that frequently frustrate an operating-room staff. Everyone in the operating arena came under the influence of the prayer, resulting in a positive outcome for all involved.

Before I became aware of my multidimensional nature and the power of love, I invested in a number of business ventures to take advantage of tax loopholes in an attempt to "get rich quick." About three years later, an energy-saving venture I had invested in with a letter of credit announced bankruptcy. Because the company was now bankrupt, the IRS disallowed my $25,000 tax credit. In the meantime, I had invested the $25,000 in an oil-leasing company. Although the company had been given a good reference by the Better Business Bureau, things began to fall apart. I read in *Newsweek* that the board of directors had been placed under indictment for fraud, as well as the area's Better Business Bureau president, who was accused of taking bribes from the company. In addition, another venture I had invested in ended in bankruptcy. So I not only had no return on my investments, I also lost the tax credit and did not have the $25,000 to pay the IRS.

It seemed that I had limited options at the time, including selling property, cashing in my retirement fund or even bankruptcy. I took the matter into prayer, focusing on trust. As a witness to my trust, I increased what I was giving to my church from 1% of my income to 5%. What transpired was most unusual. After notifying me of the disallowance, the IRS misplaced my file and therefore could not bill me. For three months the file remained lost. Toward the end of that period a commercial banking agent invited herself to my office to go over my finances to see if her bank could be of service. As a result of her visit, the bank consolidated all my debts into one note and arranged a comfortable repayment schedule. Then the IRS found my file. When they finally billed me, I was able to pay.

Thus far I have been describing experiences of supplicative prayer, which involves asking for something based on the perception or experience of a need. As we have discussed, another form is affirmative prayer. There exists in the higher energies of love the solution to all problems that honors the highest good of everyone. The solution already exists in pre-physical energy form, including the energy for the manifestation of all the things needed in the physical world. All we need to do is accept it. Using affirmative prayer acknowledges what already exists and aligns our own energies with it to receive.

For example, if we are dealing with a prosperity issue, the following affirmation is useful, "I am the presence of the great prosperity of God."[33] If the issue is health, "I am the presence of the perfect health of God." If we are tempted to be upset, "I am the presence of the peace of God." If we feel we lack love and trust, "I trust my brother with whom I am one" (ACIM W-P I.181),[17] and "I am the presence of God loving everyone (or someone). God is present in everyone (or someone) loving me." I have found the latter prayer to be a particularly powerful all-purpose affirmation. We may also use intercessory affirmations such as, "I am the presence of the perfect health of God or the perfect prosperity of God in so-and-so." In addition to using words, we may also use visualization as a form of affirmative prayer. We may visualize the goal already accomplished, allowing ourselves to accept its emotional essence through the use of the imagination.

As we release more fear and advance in our awareness, we can evolve into a higher form of prayer, which is simply to focus on love, asking for nothing, realizing that in the experience of love we already have everything. In love is total joy, the emotional essence of everything. In opening up to that joy, "needs" on the material plane are automatically and spontaneously met. This form of prayer is a state of communion where we simply acknowledge love and gratitude to God. In this state we have an energy exchange in which we reap the experience of oneness with the Creator. As we walk about between formal prayer periods, we commune with God by seeing and loving God in everyone and everything. However, the supplicative and affirmative forms of prayer may be helpful in removing subconscious blocks to the acceptance of love and change in our lives.

There is an action component of prayer as well. The way we live our lives is witness to what we hold in consciousness (our faith). As we change our consciousness we change our lives. For example, in my own experience, I had reached the point of having my debts under control and living comfortably without financial stress, but there was no extra money. After the bills were paid, we had nothing left for other useful activities, including travel or other extras. I had reached the point in my spiritual life where I was into affirmative prayer, so I spent a lot of time affirming and visualizing prosperity. But I seemed to be stuck, so in a supplicative prayer I asked for a solution to the problem. Shortly thereafter, I had an informative dream in which I saw myself in a bulldozer trying to extend a highway through a thick forest. The forest was resistant, and progress had slowed to a stand-still. Then I was lifted above the forest and roadway until I could see that another highway already existed; it skirted the forest, unobstructed, to my destination. Somehow I had missed seeing it curving off to the right. So I dropped back down and completed my journey. The next day as I was contemplating this dream in reference to my financial dilemma, I received in the mail a publication containing a long feature article on tithing. Many anecdotal experiences were cited in which individuals had transformed their finances by tithing. I knew immediately what the dream meant. I was trying to affirm my way into prosperity but the path already existed. I had excluded the essential ingredient—right action. My actions were not a witness to the faith I wanted and needed.

A tithe by definition is the giving of ten per cent of one's income, in this case for spiritual purposes. I had always thought that when I became more prosperous I would tithe. But that thought of lack perpetuated lack. It would have been a long wait. Instead I began to live a different consciousness, tithing as if I could afford it. Ten percent came off the top of my paycheck as soon as it came in. Then, to my amazement, my income unexpectedly doubled in a period of approximately three months. Now I could afford to tithe.

Prayer, like our thoughts, affects not only people, but also inanimate things. I purchased a car and was quite pleased with its quiet, smooth ride. After about two days the brake pedal started to stick. Whenever I stopped I would have to lean over and pull up the pedal manually. No matter what I did the brake continued to stick. I was faced with the inconvenience of having to take the car across town to be serviced by the dealer. Then I remembered that God was the greatest mechanic in the universe. So that night I took the matter into prayer. The next morning I tested the brake and it worked. It never stuck again.

About a year later a loud clanging rattle developed in the exhaust system. A bracket must have worked loose, and the muffler or exhaust pipe was hitting against the chassis with every minor bump. Again, the inconvenience of taking the car to the dealer did not seem to be for my highest good, although I realized that it eventually might be necessary. At this point I was into affirmative prayer, so I began to affirm the perfection of God in the car. Focusing on the car with gratitude, I emotionally ignored what my ears were hearing and pretended the car was in perfect condition. I reached for the emotional experience of a brand-new car. On the third day of this activity, my wife, Anne, and I were scheduled to take a short trip. As we drove off, the car remained silent. I hadn't mentioned what I had been doing, so before I said anything I purposely hit all the pot holes in our neighborhood to test the car. The rattle didn't return. The car drove as quietly and smoothly as when it was new, and it never rattled again. When I shared with Anne what I had been doing, she said that she had noticed the change and had assumed I had taken the car in for service.

These small experiences may seem frivolous, but there is no problem in our lives, no matter how small, that love will not correct if we are willing.

There is a tendency in the scientific community to dismiss accounts such as these as anecdotal and thus invalid as evidence. To do so is a mistake. By definition an anecdote is the account of a little known fact or happening. Large case studies are made up of numerous anecdotes. Even randomized, double-blind studies are collections of many anecdotes. If science is to go beyond itself and explore new ground, it must look at evidence that is beyond the experience of large randomized studies. Then it can use this new information to develop and fund large prospective or retrospective studies to gather together a body of evidence upon which our culture can rely in order to make good decisions. We must not disparage the anecdote; it is an important first step and often may be the only step available. If the established scientific community does not respond, it may be that the grass-root anecdotal experiences of the general public will direct the choices of our culture for its own good.

Science disparages the anecdote in an attempt to protect us against fraud. Too often this disparaging of the anecdote comes from a need to be "right" and an unwillingness to change perceptions and shift to a new paradigm. The randomized, double-blind study can be a useful reality check if its design is based on true premises; otherwise it will truly be doubly blind, as when the blind lead the blind. Such a study must take into account the power of the mind even at the unconscious level. Rather than attempt to separate effect from consciousness, the design must allow for the effect of consciousness. For example, the study must take into account the faiths of the physician and client. The placebo effect is a real effect we want to utilize. In fact, in a sense, every effect is a placebo effect, even those that can be defined and described molecularly. The activity of molecules is not independent of consciousness. Consciousness is cause.

The premise that science has operated on in the past is that there is an objective reality independent of consciousness, that consciousness is a secondary phenomenon operative only in the limited confines of the rules of that objective reality. In fact, there is no objective reality independent of consciousness. Physical reality is a subjective experience. This understanding must be incorporated into the design of scientific studies if science is to be of most benefit in guiding us to our fullest potential for benevolent dominion over our experience.

Everyone has experienced what appears to be unanswered prayers. Yet according to mystical sources, all prayers are answered; we just don't recognize the answers or are unable to accept them at the moment. Most of us have also had the experience of wanting something, but, when we get it, we're afraid of it, or it seems to cause problems that result in fear. Also, there are often secondary gains to an illness or a negative situation that we may not be able to release. It is love that answers prayer, and love does not change a situation if that change would increase our fear beyond our ability to deal with it appropriately.

The problem might also be that we are hanging on to conscious or unconscious guilt, which contains the perception that we don't deserve good things in our lives. If we feel undeserving, we will be uncomfortable when we experience something good.

Anger is an attempt to repress fear and guilt. If we hold on to it, the unhealed guilt behind it will block the answer to prayer. Thus forgiveness is essential if we are to experience answered prayers. Another way of expressing this is to say that a willingness to love unconditionally is necessary for the complete experience of having our prayers answered. This does not mean that at a given moment we have to feel unconditional love, but there must be some willingness to love. Through our little bit of willingness, love then expresses for our good.

Forgiveness is the letting go of guilt, fear, anger or grief, allowing them to be replaced by love. This step always involves a change in perception. True forgiveness, like the love that makes it possible, is unconditional. No penance or change is required. The other person does not have to change or apologize, no matter what was done or not done. To give unconditional love is to love as if you have no past at all with that person; to love as if no injury or abuse had occurred; to see the person as totally innocent no matter what he is doing or has done. True forgiveness is not pardon but acquittal.

Since love and joy are synonymous, to place no conditions on love is to open to unconditional happiness. If we release the conditions we think are required for happiness and open up to experiencing what already exists within, not waiting for change, the energy with the power to change will come forth, producing a reflection of happiness in the events of our lives. As we open to the wisdom of this love, we see through the vision of reality, and forgiveness becomes a spontaneous experience. As I have said, this love must be directed toward everyone, including ourselves.

It is too much to expect at this point that we will be able to spontaneously feel this level of love, nor can we generate it when we don't feel it. It is simply enough for us to become willing to feel it. Love already exists beyond our awareness, and it operates through our willingness. We may first experience it when we realize that it is operating around us, changing events, without our conscious participation. Or our first experience of it may occur as a spontaneous shift in our feelings before external change is seen. We may simply feel love where we once felt hate. Of course, our words and actions will reflect this new feeling as will the changes in the world around us.

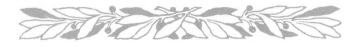

Chapter 8

HOOKS AND SNARES

Everyone desires to be happy. The hooks and snares that keep us from satisfying that desire are usually the very things we think will make us happy. No one would purposely allow himself to be hooked on unhappiness, but the hook has made it look, smell and feel like the real thing.

A salesman friend shared with me this story: "God decided to give those who made it to Heaven a choice of staying or going to hell. In case they were curious about the alternative, he gave them a chance to visit hell first. The situation was appropriately explained by St. Peter to the next arrival, who thought, 'Oh what the hell, I think I'll go down and check it out.' He no sooner had the thought than he found himself being led on a tour of hell by the devil. What he saw amazed him: a beautiful country club with fantastic golf courses, tennis courts, pools, dining facilities, entertainment and beautiful people. He began to think that all the bad press about hell must have been misguided. When he returned to Heaven, he asked for a tour there before he made his decision. He was shown around another country-club-like setting, but it wasn't as attractive or as exciting as the one he had visited in hell, so he decided he wanted hell. As soon as he had the thought, he found himself chained to a bare concrete wall in a hot, smelly dungeon surrounded by all sorts of indescribable horrors, not the least of which were the flames licking at his feet. Standing nearby was the devil, who did not at all resemble the well-spoken man in the business suit who led him on his tour of hell. 'I don't understand,' our man said. 'Just a few moments ago you were showing me this fantastic country club and now this. There must be some mistake.' Without hesitation the devil responded, 'Yes, but then you were just a prospect.'"

I made some references to hooks and snares in earlier discussion of attempts at self-definition. All hooks take on some form of special-ness. Someone, something or some event is singled out as special. They relate to us and we relate to them in a special way. I will explain in more detail what the hooks and snares look like, how they work and why we have them. Then you might be able to recognize them, unhook yourself and avoid being hooked again.

As the mind of the child-to-be focuses its energy into the earth realm to prepare for the incarnation, its awareness, as discussed in Chapter 5, is not limited to the energy patterns of the body and the body's nervous system. Thus the incoming individual is directly (telepathically) aware most immediately of the energy patterns (the thoughts and feelings) of the mother and immediate family, then the culture.

Perceptions and feelings of rejection and separation are inherent in our cultural experience at this time. For example, if the mother is not happy about having a baby or is ambivalent about it, the incarnating mind is aware of her attitude. The message received is: "I am not want-ed; I am unworthy; I am rejected, thus rejectable." The child-to-be begins to feel separated from the parent-to-be.

I had one patient who got in touch with the fact that she had been depressed since birth. The family's heart had been set on a boy, so her appearance was greeted with disappointment. Since her awareness was not limited to the physical brain, she felt the full impact of this nega-tive emotion and thus felt rejected. This feeling was reinforced at both conscious and unconscious levels as she grew.

As a child learns to use the brain and communicate through the body's senses, usually he or she becomes unaware of the expanded nature of the mind. Yet the child is still influenced by thoughts and feelings of which it is unaware, as well as by those that are verbalized or carried out as actions.

Helen Schucman[113] remembered as a toddler feeling happy and good about herself. One day her father stood in the doorway of her room looking at her, saying nothing. All of a sudden the feeling of being ugly overwhelmed her, and stayed with her. As she grew older, she became somewhat unattractive, matching her new perception of herself. This perception had been communicated to her through the unconscious realm of the mind, where there are no hidden thoughts or feelings, as her father, seeing her through the cloud of his own negativity, saw her as ugly. Her awareness of the significance of this event came through a spontaneous "flash back" when she became open to healing.

The rejection experience may be silent, subtle or overt. It may be camouflaged in civility or overtly abusive. It may be unavoidable, as when a new baby diverts the attention of the mother from the older child. Or it may result from the illness or death of a parent or some other important person in the child's life. Many other circumstances may be involved in which the child loses the attention of someone who has played an important role in his or her life.

Another subtle form of rejection is found simply in the impatient response of a worried, hassled parent. More overtly, it may occur in the form of "justified" wrath. Anytime someone is angry (impatient, frustrated, annoyed, irritated) with us, we receive the message of rejection. The child who has been put to bed but longs for one more contact with the loved parent calls out. The parent, tired after a busy day and yearning for a few moments of rest, feels threatened and in desperation calls back impatiently, "What!" The child feels the anger energy through his expanded unconscious and hears it in the parent's tone of voice. The message is rejection. That message is associated with feelings of guilt and fear. This does not mean the parent does not deserve time alone; the problem is in the emotional energy of the response, not the form of the response, although the emotional energy may determine the form. Such episodes tend to occur over and over again in a child's life.

Another subtle form of "betrayal" comes when the integrity of the child is rejected by a benevolent but overly strict, controlling parent. The child gets the message that he or she is not competent to make decisions or to adequately and safely express himself or herself verbally or through actions. On the other hand, lack of attention in the form of appropriate guidance may teach the child that he or she is unworthy. These lessons may also be taught in less benevolent, more overtly neglectful or critical and abusive ways, with increasingly severe effects.

The child may also be negatively impacted by negative behavior not necessarily directed at him or her. The perception is: "What happens to another may happen to me." Or: "What someone else does I have the potential of doing." We tend, to some extent, to identify with all life forms, but most closely with humans and then even more closely with those in our immediate family and environment. Thus our parents' negative experiences may teach us that whatever happened to them can happen to us, or that what they do we will do also. As we identify with our parents, we in a sense become extensions of them, and we tend to absorb their pain and their perceptions.

An example of this is the case of a woman who grew up in a large family from which her father was frequently absent. Her mother was insecure and felt overwhelmed. The household was in chaos. As an older daughter, some of the responsibility for order fell upon her shoulders. Eventually she married and became the mother of two young children. When her husband was away on business she would begin to feel overwhelmed, anxious and irritable. In other words, she would fall apart, just like her mother. She had absorbed her mother's pain and perceptions.

These negative interfaces with the world around us tend to occur to some degree in all areas of human experience, including intellectual/professional, social, moral, material/financial and physical. Rejection experienced in one area may cause feelings of inadequacy to spill over into another, resulting in the acceptance of negative perceptions about oneself in those areas as well. We attempt to repress these negative feelings and these perceptions, by hiding them first from the world and then from ourselves. These feelings and perceptions become the secret self.

We attempt to hide from this secret self and thus repress these feelings and perceptions by making ourselves what we secretly believe we are not. Our family, peers and culture teach us what and how we have to be in order to avoid rejection. Thus we are validated when we meet certain cultural standards and win the acceptance of others. These standards, this perfect person, form the ego ideal. If we are a certain way, we will feel worthy—in other words, less guilty. This temporary release from guilt causes us to feel temporarily happy. Unaware of our true nature, we attempt to sustain the ego ideal to maintain happiness. The result is a facade self (the ego facade), which we present to ourselves and the world. The people, things and events that we think will make this facade look like the ego ideal become special to us, and we become attached to and dependent on them.

This method of repression is what I call substitution. The facade is a substitute for what we truly are, and the things, people and events that make up the ego ideal are substitutes for what we really want. These substitutes become the hooks and snares that actually keep us from true happiness.

The happiness these substitutes seem to provide is false and leads only to disappointment and more fear and guilt. No real happiness can be found in the ego ideal, even if the ego ideal were obtainable by substitution. However, in spite of everything the individual does to make the ego ideal possible, including his attempts to control others, failure is inevitable because the individual really has faith in the secret self. Thus the secret self is what ultimately becomes manifest and the facade begins to break down. The extent of the breakdown depends on the degree of belief in this hidden self. If the dominant belief (in other words, our faith) is that we are inadequate, then that is what will become manifest. To repeat what I discussed in Chapter 6, if the dominant energy is guilt, then we will experience guilt's punishment. If the dominant energy is fear, the world will become frightening. If the dominant energy is anger, the guilt hidden behind it will produce an angry world. If the dominant energy is grief, then we will attract something over which to grieve.

As the facade self begins to fall apart because the ego ideal is unrealized, the fear and guilt it was designed to repress begin to increase and to surface. This usually leads to more frantic attempts at substitution and to other forms of repression.

The irony of the situation is that behind the negative emotions we attempt to repress is what we really want: the unaltered love and joy that is our life force continually expressed through us, as us, from God. This is the original, unaltered state of our emotions. It is this life force of emotional energy that gives us consciousness, awareness and the capacity to think; it beats our heart and gives us breath; it is the energy that manifests the body and the things and events of our lives. This energy can be altered by the mind's negative perceptions, and in its altered form we know it as fear and guilt. As we attempt to repress fear and guilt, we repress the emotional energy that gives us life and creative power. And, as I have said, what we really desire, the love and joy hidden behind the fear and guilt, is also repressed. If we could completely repress our emotions, we would cease to exist, but that is not possible. The emotional energy builds up until it explodes forth, just as our attempt to hold our breath ends in a gasp for air.

To avoid feeling these painful emotions and yet allow our emotional energy to flow, we disguise fear and guilt and express them in a form that seems to be more acceptable (less painful). The disguised form, however, is still negative. Guilt is translated into anger and thus expressed by accepting the false perception that someone else is at fault; that someone else is responsible for an unpleasant circumstance; that "someone/something else has power over me, so I am not responsible." This process is called projection. Guilt is projected as anger toward something outside of self.

How this process is managed depends most importantly on how the individual is programmed in the first few years of life. This results in characteristic behavior patterns or patterns of projection.

If the parent has been overly controlling and repressive in either an over-protective or overtly abusive way, the child may become programmed to believe that he or she will be controlled or, in the more severe scenario, victimized. He also may learn that to express anger or other emotions is dangerous.

This person will be more passive in his or her expression of anger—in other words, passive-aggressive. The anger is expressed as blaming and complaining, usually behind the back of the perceived villain. If the anger is expressed directly, it is usually done with caution and with little hope of bringing about change. The primary reason for blaming and complaining is to release emotional pressure by altering the energy of guilt and expressing it as anger. The individual actually needs something or someone to blame and complain about in order to disguise guilt. A sense of relief follows as the pain of guilt is temporarily repressed and the altered emotional life force is converted into and expressed as anger. This is the attraction to gossiping and criticism. In addition to serving as an emotional release valve, the act of putting someone else down (making him or her seem less worthy) seems to establish a higher level of self-worth.

The traits we are most likely to complain about in another are those that reflect our hated secret self. The other person, in this case, serves as an unconscious reminder of what we hate in ourselves. As this self-hatred (guilt) begins to surface, we translate it into anger toward the one who reminds us of our own perceived inadequacies. Anger may also be felt toward someone we envy, as their success reminds us of our perceived failure.

This type of individual usually believes, consciously or unconsciously, that he or she will be controlled or victimized, meaning that he will attract people with a tendency to control or victimize. As stated, the victim experience serves the need to blame and complain by providing something about which blaming and complaining seems to be justified.

Another way we attempt to release guilt is to translate it into pain and suffering. Suffering seems to temporarily appease the feelings of guilt. This leads to moaning and groaning, which is often combined with some degree of blaming and complaining. If an individual's parents have been overly punishing, his passive-aggressive behavior is more likely to take on this masochistic pattern. In the pure masochist there is little blaming of anyone other than oneself.

If moaning and groaning is not part of the ego ideal, an individual prone to pain and suffering may adopt an attitude of grin and bear it. This is the martyr complex. As with the moaner and groaner, this perception will unconsciously attract individuals likely to contribute to the experience of suffering.

If the ego ideal does not require a grin, but still does not allow blaming and complaining, the individual may exhibit a grit-and-bear-it pattern. In this case, the ego ideal does not allow for the expression of much emotion. He or she is likely to be emotionally withdrawn, going through life with stoic determination. The emotional withdrawal, which arises primarily for self-protection, may also result from the passive expression of anger in an attempt to punish and manipulate others in order to have them conform to the needs of the ego facade.

If an individual's early childhood has included permissiveness as well as rejection, a different mode of expressing negative emotions may evolve. In this situation, periods of benevolence may be followed by what the child perceives as betrayal; or the permissive atmosphere may be the result of indifferent neglect by an otherwise critical or abusive parent or other adults. In this case the individual may be less fearful of expressing his anger. Also, if the parent has been aggressive in his or her relationship with others, as well as permissive or neglectful toward the child, the child is likely to become aggressive. In other words, as previously discussed, children tend to model themselves after the behavioral characteristics of the parent if they perceive it is safe to do so, even if they don't like those characteristics. The unconscious belief becomes, "They are like that, so I will be like that, too." This behavior becomes part of the secret self. The secret perception is, "I am a villain." For some people, aggressive behavior may become part of the consciously sought ego ideal, just as passive behavior is the ideal for others.

In these situations, the individual will become what I call active-aggressive. The anger is expressed more overtly, with the intent to cause suffering to control and effect change in others. This individual "slashes and kills," at least figuratively, by verbal abuse, or through manipulation of situations, if not by physical violence. Blaming may also be part of the pattern if it is needed by the ego ideal to justify the slash-and-kill behavior.

If being a villain is not part of the ego ideal, the individual may unconsciously learn to justify slashing and killing by finding injustices to correct and a perpetrator of injustice to slash and kill. This individual goes on a search-and-rescue mission to seek out a villain-victim situation. In rescuing the victim, the villain can be justifiably slashed and killed, and the emotional energy of guilt is released as righteous wrath. This is the Robin Hood complex. If a villain-victim combination is not "legitimately" found, the individual is likely to imagine one and will try to convince someone he is a victim in need of rescue. This type of motivation is present in many people who become involved in otherwise worthy causes. However, things done out of anger usually produce angry results.

Transference to any available target for projection may occur. If an actual "villain" is not available or if it is considered unsafe to direct anger toward the perceived real villain, an alternate will unconsciously be sought and found.

Patterns of Projection

Passive-Aggressive	Blame and complain.
	Moan and groan.
	Grin and bear it.
	Grit and bear it.
Active-Aggressive	Slash and kill.
	Search and rescue.

An individual may switch modes of expressing negative emotions depending on which behavior is considered safe or vital for a particular set of circumstances. For example, someone could be passive-aggressive at work, but active-aggressive at home.

It is important to realize that until we have become awakened to these dynamics we will be controlled by negative emotional needs, and the urgency to express them in these modes may be as great and uncontrollable as the need to breathe. Thus compassion rather than criticism is the enlightened response to those who exhibit passive-aggressive or active-aggressive behavior, whether the individual is one-self or someone else.

If we follow the formula with a willingness to forgive and love, healing will take place and the dynamic will change.

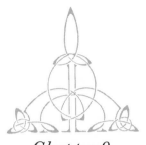

Chapter 9

SPECIAL HATE
RELATIONSHIPS

As I have discussed, the passive-aggressive blamer and complainer, moaner and groaner, etc. have been programmed to believe that they will be victimized. In addition to having this expectation, such people also need to be victimized to provide a reason to blame and complain or moan and groan. These factors result in the unconscious attraction of the elements needed for the manifestation of victimhood. On the other hand the active-aggressive has been programmed to believe he or she is a slasher and killer, and has a need to slash and kill.

These unconscious energies reach out into the collective energy field of consciousness, where they meet and mesh with other energies until agreeing combinations are formed. These energy combinations then bring individuals together in an appropriate situation matching their predominant belief systems and needs. This situation will be the playing out of what may be called a special hate relationship.

Special hate relationships can be obvious or subtle, yet the basic emotional energy dynamics are always the same. Have you ever enjoyed gossiping or being critical of people or institutions? Have you ever had a sense of relief at telling someone off? In such experiences, those persons or institutions served a special purpose: they served as objects to satisfy the need to express anger, and that expression of anger brought about an immediate sense of relief. Have you ever known people in a relationship at work, in a marriage or in some other social setting who were always in conflict, and yet the combatants stayed together or kept coming back together? Such is the special hate relationship to which both participants are unconsciously attracted and without which they would not be "happy." They have an unconscious need to hate, to let off steam, so that their feelings of fear and guilt can be soothed and their self-hate can be temporarily diverted.

For illustration I will share examples I have observed. The names and circumstances have been altered somewhat for the sake of anonymity.

Jack was the leader of a group activity. His barely repressed perception of himself was that he was a failure—not that the world would have judged him as such, based on what he had accomplished in his life. However, his accomplishments were not sufficient to appease his repressed feelings of guilt and fear. He felt incompetent and irresponsible. His guilt (self hate) was quite strong and needed expression. In other words, he needed to be angry. Because of the nature of his childhood programming he was not afraid to express his anger.

Jack's perception of his own incompetence was an unconscious thought-energy pattern that vibrated through his omnipresent mind and attracted someone with a similar, complimentary pattern that meshed with his unconscious need to project. That person turned out to be Jane, who also had a self-perception of incompetence. But her perception was not as repressed. Being a moaner and groaner, she publicly acknowledged that she could never do anything right. Because of her early childhood programming she didn't feel free to actively express anger but rather needed to release the emotional energy of guilt through suffering. In her case the suffering in part took the form of verbal self-abuse. Consciously she feared the judgment of others; thus she publicly expressed anger toward herself, hoping this would lessen criticism from others by causing them to take pity on her. Unconsciously, however, she needed to be attacked by others so she could suffer more. Yet like all attempts to escape feelings of guilt by misthinking, it didn't work. The pain increased, and so did failure, personal ridicule and suffering.

The unconscious energies of these two manifested the synchronicities that brought them together in the same organization, where they unconsciously recognized each other. Without realizing why, Jack became irritated in her presence. She was beginning to remind him of his own secret self. In like manner, Jane became nervous in Jack's presence. When she was given some responsibilities in the organization, Jane failed to carry them out successfully. What Jack had unconsciously suspected, he could now consciously see. He went into a rage, verbally attacking Jane, blaming her and complaining about her to others. She accepted the attack, and cowered in self-pity while moaning and groaning. Now she obviously had good reason to moan and groan, for the group leader had verbally beat her up in front of everyone. Moaning and groaning alone was not sufficiently satisfying, so she made some attempt at relief by blaming and complaining about the lack of sympathy, understanding and help from Jack.

The relationship was like ongoing warfare, yet neither party would release him or herself. They needed each other. Jack needed to slash and kill, and Jane needed to moan and groan. However, what may be experienced in the moment as relief does not always provide what is desired—quite the contrary. In this situation, mutual misery increased. Jack's misthoughts and negative behavior intensified his feelings of guilt, which in turn intensified his anger and fear. And the same dynamic operated for Jane. Furthermore, they unconsciously experienced each other's feelings as their own. Jane's increasing depression intensified Jack's sadness and disappointment in himself, and vice versa. A mutually shared, self-perpetuating and increasing negative energy dynamic was set into motion.

The solution to this problem could have been reached by not taking the bait. If Jack had been more self-aware, at his first feelings of irritation with Jane he would have realized that he was feeling guilty about being irritated. He wouldn't deny either feeling but would embrace them both. Nor would he let his feelings control him, but rather would take dominion over them by acknowledging that he would prefer to feel another way. He would begin to affirm thoughts that were compatible with the feelings he would prefer to have. He could use prayer and meditation to release the negative emotions and their perceptions. As Jane began to act out her negative beliefs about herself, Jack would again have to go through the process and look for another way to interrelate with her.

Jane would begin to be unconsciously impacted by the energy of love that Jack was directing to her and would begin to feel better about herself. If she stumbled, Jack would help her in a way that would allow her to develop more confidence in herself. He would focus on his trust in her and affirm her perfection and success, and he could also visualize her success. Jane would unconsciously pick up these thought forms, feel more confidence and begin to experience more success.

Depending on how intense and deep Jack's fear was, he might not at first feel much love for or trust in Jane. He would have to fake it for a while. But as he continued to focus on his intent to love, he would eventually begin to feel spontaneous good feelings toward Jane. These would be his true feelings, his unaltered life force through which he would experience his own release from fear and his own true happiness and success.

As Jane began to feel better, Jack would unconsciously receive her joyous energy, which would be added to his own. Thus both would become increasingly happy. Jane would be successful in completing her project. And both would begin to feel good about each other and enjoy working together. Because they had begun to experience the energy of love, their mutual accomplishments would become more and more successful and rewarding.

What was once a special hate relationship would become an unconditionally loving relationship. The essential ingredient of this now Holy relationship is the love that comes through a willingness to forgive: to forgive oneself for one's own perceived failures and to forgive the other person for his or her failures. In forgiveness is the willingness to see the perfection in others and in oneself, letting go of what may have occurred in the past—years ago, last year, yesterday or even in the last millisecond.

To allow this shift to occur one must let go of the immediately gratifying experience of expressing anger in an attempt to be rid of the pain of guilt. Not to let go is to continue being hooked by more guilt.

Either member of a special hate relationship may bring enlightenment to it. If it had been Jane, at the first fear-thought of failure, she would have affirmed her abilities in a positive way and used prayer and meditation for healing. In the face of Jack's negative behavior, she would have approached him with love, which would have eased his fears, allowing a positive change to occur in their relationship.

No matter how impossible the situation might seem, any relationship can be healed. Free will operates, however. If either person had been unwilling to release guilt and anger, he or she could have refused what was offered from the other and have left the relationship. Fear cannot survive in the presence of love; so if one person expressed love, the energy of mutual negative attraction would no longer be present, and the relationship would no longer serve the need of the one not ready to accept love.

I have already discussed the power of trust in dire circumstances. I will relate another real life situation. Judith Skutch,[108] who lived in a large American city, heard a news report of a young woman who had been sexually assaulted and murdered on the subway that morning. Judith thought about the episode often during the day and began to experience fear for her own safety, particularly since she was planning to use the same subway line later that evening to attend a meeting. Her fear-thoughts were like radio waves going out into the collective energy of consciousness where they were received by the unconscious aspect of someone tuned to this pattern—in other words, someone who needed to attack. In this case that person was someone who had experienced deprivation and was dealing with the energy of repressed guilt over his failure to be in a better financial situation. He needed an object for projection, someone at whom to be angry. That object would be a person economically and educationally much better off. The contrast would be a reminder of his own failings and would provide a perfect object for projection. Judith fit the role of that special person. We may also assume that this person was neglected or abused by his mother, and he had transfered his anger at his mother toward all women.

The energies of the unconscious mingled and joined together in manifesting the synchronicities that brought this man together with Judith in a subway car, alone except for two other men of similar mind-set who were with him. As Judith observed the three men entering the car, her judgment was that they were the types who might carry out an attack such as the one she had read about. Her fears increased; thus she became increasingly vulnerable to attack. Looking at her, the men seemed to be discussing her fate. Then the man in question stood up and began to walk toward her. In addition to her own perceptions, Judith was unconsciously receiving and agreeing with his thought-energy, which was focused on the idea of attack. She sensed he was not just after her purse. As her fear increased, she remembered something. She closed her eyes and prayed, asking to see the situation another way. Now willing to love, she opened her eyes and saw before her a being of such beauty that she began to smile. In her willingness to feel love for him, she was actually being given a vision of his Higher Nature. The dominant energy of her mind no longer agreed with the images of attack and fear. Instead, love was directed toward the would-be attacker. At first, the effect of this new high frequency energy on the consciousness of the man was confusion. He seemed to be stunned. Then he backed away and sat down. The three men sat in silence. When the subway car finally stopped, Judith's purse fell to the floor. The man who had planned to attack her got up, handed her the purse and said, "Have a good day, ma'am." Then the three men left the car.

What was to have been the acting out of a special hate relationship became in an instant an unconditional love relationship. Often love is not consciously experienced in the early moments of a crisis, but if one expresses a willingness to love, love will enter through the unconscious and bring about change. In other words, one does not have to be afraid of fear. Willingness is all that is necessary for love to express and change a situation.

Once one becomes aware of the dynamic of projection in special hate relationships, it is easy to spot it happening between others. The next step is to realize when it is happening to us. Once I was working with someone similar to Jack. I was conducting a meeting at which he was present that had gone ten minutes beyond the scheduled time for ending. Knowing how impatient this individual was (I will call him Bob), I became nervous that he would be critical. Of course, I was putting out the thought form that would help create that outcome. Bob was not only receptive to the thought because of his need to project, but he had already begun to put his own energy into it. Sure enough, after I closed the meeting he got up and delivered a slash-and-kill lecture on incompetency, irresponsibility and the inability to end a meeting on time. In doing so, he overlooked the fact that he had arrived at that same meeting twenty minutes late.

Sometimes we attract criticism by fearing it, which is the same thing as expecting it. There are many people who need to criticize and will be attracted to us to play out that role. As I became more self-vigilant, I became aware that I was seldom criticized unless I expected it. This is not to say that we always attract the criticisms and would-be assaults that occur. Some people's need to project is so great they will use any convenient target, whether there is an invitation or not. Sometimes the contrast between the appearance of innocence in another and the self-perception of guilt stirs even more guilt, and the innocent become the target. (The word "innocent" is used here figuratively, for in fact everyone is innocent.) Remember, however, if one holds his peace and focuses on love and trust, no harm can come, and the slasher and killer or blamer and complainer will have to retreat.

The final step for me was to realize when I was projecting onto others. In one group with which I was working on a project, I began to find Mary's presence very irritating. She was a talkative, clinging and needy person whose presence and harebrained ideas were distracting and delaying. My feelings of irritation were compounded by the guilt I felt at not feeling love and compassion for her. I knew the truth intellectually but was not able to experience it emotionally. So I faked it. I meditated and prayed for the ability to love her. What came to me in meditation was a memory of a long-ago event that had nothing to do with this person and for which I felt much guilt. It was an upsetting memory, and my guilt over it stayed with me for about three days. On the third day, while reading *A Course in Miracles*,[17] it suddenly, spontaneously lifted. The next day Mary showed up and wanted to meet with me. I was amazed that when we met I no longer had those unnerving, irritated feelings. I was able to listen to her in peace. That was the last time I saw her, because she chose to go on to other things. When I released guilt, her neediness was no longer a source of irritation. Her behavior and energy apparently had unconsciously reminded me of a part of myself that I hated. The self-hate emerged as anger toward her. When it was healed, her unconscious negative attraction to me was gone. That she left at that point was no accident.

In a similar situation, I found myself having difficulty loving Bill. In this case I prayed with great intensity for the ability to love. The next time I saw him I was overwhelmed by feelings of love and compassion for him that have never left. Bill was able to accept this higher energy, and he stayed in my life. I am glad he did, for I still rejoice when I see him. In this case, the change occurred without a memory or awareness of repressed feelings.

Chapter 10

SPECIAL LOVE
RELATIONSHIPS

E arlier I discussed some of my own experiences with the special
love relationship. For emphasis I will repeat some of that information in this chapter and add more.

We become attached to the things and people that make up the
image of the ego ideal, for without them the ego facade would fall
apart. The emperor would realize he wasn't wearing any clothes and
feel ashamed. We become dependent on these special things and people to the point that we feel that we cannot do without them. As long
as we are hopeful of getting the desired person or thing, or perceive
that we have it, we feel less fear and guilt. Temporarily successful in
using the special love relationship to validate self as worthy and thus
unaware of the repressed guilt that created the need for the relationship, we seem to feel love and joy. This feeling of false love is directed
toward that special person or thing. What we have perceived as love is
really hate in disguise—hatred of self. If the disguise breaks down, the
special love is lost and its true nature is exposed. Guilt surfaces and is
projected as anger toward the special person. This is why as an adolescent and young adult I believed that the flip side of love was hate. This
is not true. The flip side of real love is joy, and there is no pain associated with it.

As discussed earlier, the ego ideal is made up of our professional and intellectual pursuits, philosophy of life and adherence to that philosophy (morality), financial and material possessions, what our physical body looks like and how it performs and our human relationships (with family, friends, acquaintances and strangers). If these components seem to work for us, we love them; if they don't work, we hate them. Either way, we make them special.

What better way to know we are worthy and to feel good about ourselves than to have another person tell us in some way that we are okay? Or better yet, to have someone tell us they like and care for us and that they want to become our friend. Still better is for someone to commit their life to us above all others. This seems to make us very special indeed. This occurs in couple relationships, marriages and other family relationships, such as parent-child. The ultimate commitment is marriage—to have someone commit to an exclusive relationship with us, to establish a home and family with us. Wife, husband and family are important aspects of the ego ideal in our culture. Yet they invariably lead to some degree of disappointment.

About half of all marriages end in divorce. Many of those that remain intact are unhappy, and most of the rest are less than completely satisfying. Many if not all of these marriages began with infatuation—the feeling of being madly in love—yet most of them wind up with elements of the special hate relationship.

This is not to say that the institution of marriage and family is bad. But if we seek it out as the source of our happiness we will be disappointed. We can, however, bring happiness to these relationships as we allow them to become tools to teach love and remove blocks to our awareness of love's presence.

In spite of such miserable statistics, most of us at one time or another wanted more than anything to have a special person make that commitment to us. In the ego-ideal family, not just any wife, husband or child will do. We are programmed by our family and culture as to what type of person will be acceptable—in other words, the type of person who will affirm that we are worthy. We become attracted to a person whose facade is a reasonable match to our ego ideal. If our facade matches their ego ideal, we have a "match made in heaven." The specifics in form of special love relationships vary from individual to individual, but the overall emotional content and outcome are always the same. Fear and guilt re-emerge and are projected as anger.

These special love relationships fail for a combination of reasons:

• The ego ideal changes
• The secret self becomes manifest and is discovered
• Inherent guilt arises from substitution
• Substitutes never work

The ego ideal is seldom static. For example a young man in college may be happy about marrying his girlfriend, who agrees to drop out of school to work, support him and raise the kids while he continues his education. After he gets his graduate degree, let's say in business administration, he becomes a rising corporate executive. His new ego ideal requires a wife who also has some advanced education and business success. He now feels he has outgrown his wife. "She hasn't kept up with me," he thinks. "She doesn't meet my needs." He meets such a woman and "falls in love"; there is a separation, then divorce. What was once a special love relationship now becomes a special hate relationship. "After all I did for him," the wife complains, "he dumped me."

Our children can also make us feel special. If the parent-child relationship is structured after the ego ideal as a substitute for happiness, we will be in for disappointment. The nature of the relationship will change because children grow and change. In one example, a father loved his son very much, and the son admired and respected his father in return. The father was a lower-level executive, a position that did not adequately serve his facade self because his ego ideal demanded more. He secretly thought of himself as a failure. Therefore the admiration and respect of his son was important to him. When the son became an adult, he too went into business, but he had more success than his father. The contrast accentuated the father's guilt about his perceived failure. As the guilt rose to the surface, the father, without realizing it, translated his feelings into anger toward the son. He began to look for things in his son's experience that he could criticize. If he couldn't find them, he unconsciously made them up and believed his fabrications to be real. The son was confused and upset by this. What had been a special love relationship was now a special hate relationship. The father's guilt was strong, so nothing the son did was good enough.

Not everyone reacts the same way. Another father who had not achieved much personal success might have taken vicarious pleasure in his son's successes because they defined him as a successful father.

Another example is the mother who wanted her son to be a doctor. Even though the son wanted to be an actor, the mother pressured her son into going to medical school. He experienced increasing frustration in the pursuit of a career he didn't want. His frustration led to anger toward his mother that he was unable to repress or change. So the relationship changed. If the son had chosen to become an actor in spite of his mother's pressure, she would have felt betrayed. Her ego ideal required her to have a doctor for a son. She might have felt that, in spite of all her work and sacrifice, her unappreciative son was throwing away the possibility of a beautiful career. She might have been unable to contain her disappointment and anger, which were really her conscious reactions to poorly repressed guilt. Once again the special love relationship would have failed and been replaced by a special hate relationship.

The ones we are closest to are the ones with whom we get the angriest, because they are the most special and are supposed to make us happy. When they don't (and they can't), guilt comes out as anger that may seem to be beyond our control.

Another reason the special love relationship fails is that, ultimately, the secret self is discovered. In a couple relationship, usually what happens is that no matter how the facades may appear, the secret self unconsciously attracts the appropriate matching secret self. For example, a victim will attract a villain so she or he can be victimized. Or a victim will attract another victim so together they can share a victimizing situation. One insecure person will attract another insecure person. One who perceives rejection will attract another. Ultimately the facade breaks down and the secret self is exposed. The victim and villain play out their blame-complain and slash-kill roles. The insecure person feels angry with the insecure companion. Each rejectee believes he or she has been rejected by the other.

For example, a man who has experienced rejection by his mother and misses that nurturing feminine energy seeks out a woman to provide it for him. One won't be enough, however, so he will seek others, but they won't provide what he really wants, either. If bound by morality to marriage and a monogamous relationship, he may still unconsciously seek this substitute mother in his work associates and friendships. However, the energy of lack and insecurity unconsciously attracts women who themselves are lacking and insecure. Although initially it appears they will be supportive, he winds up being rejected or at best having to support the women, who are also in need. Until the unconscious energy dynamic has been healed, this scenario will be repeated again and again.

A specific example of the mutual rejection dynamic occurred in the case of a man who, at an early age, had been rejected by his mother, although not consciously on her part. She had become depressed and was unable to respond to his need for companionship and affection. Perceiving rejection, the son felt hurt and angry. The pain was so great it was almost immediately repressed and the young lad attempted to distract himself in the various activities of life. As he matured into adulthood he found himself repeatedly falling into relationships with women whom he placed on a maternal pedestal, but in the end he was always rejected. Finally he bonded with a woman at work. She was older, and he saw her as wiser and more experienced. He placed her in a role of mentor, which was, subconsciously, the role of mother. The woman was a first child. Her mother had been very young and the child was raised by her grandmother. When the mother's circumstances improved, she had more children, whom she raised herself, but she never took back her first child. The first child was crushed and as a result felt the ongoing experience of rejection. In her relationship with the man in question, her own fear of rejection caused hostile behavior in the work situation to such an extent that the man had to give her an ultimatum: change your behavior or leave the work relationship. She of course saw this as another rejection and left angrily. The man was crushed by both her initial behavior and her angry exodus from his life. He experienced all over again the emotions of his childhood experience. These two people unconsciously attracted each other, and their repressed emotions brought about the events and interactions that turned their special love relationship into a special hate relationship as they both felt rejected by the other. When the man sought counsel, this dynamic was pointed out to him and healing began. For him, the cycle was finally interrupted.

The manifestation of rejection by the secret self may occur in one area exclusive of others, depending upon the specifics of an individual's hidden beliefs. For example, a businessman may be able to maintain a successful marriage but will experience repeated rejection and sabotage in his business.

The failure of special relationships may switch from one area to another. Betty was successful at work as long as her personal relationships were in shambles. When she had a temporarily successful personal relationship, her business would fail. This cycle repeated itself several times before she discovered in counseling that her repressed guilt would not permit her to be successful in two major areas of her life at the same time.

Sometimes the secret self of one person contaminates the facade of the other. If a man has a self-perception of inadequacy, he may also feel that his possessions are inadequate. After establishing a relationship, he thinks there is something wrong with his mate because she loves him (she is his now and is contaminated by his own perception). He becomes irritated because he no longer sees her as matching the ego ideal that would make him whole.

When an insecure person begins to see through the facade of confidence of an insecure person he has attracted, he feels irritation because the other person reminds him of himself. Guilt surfaces and is immediately translated into anger, which he has to express in some form. Of course his anger confirms the other person's feelings of insecurity, causing guilt to surface in that person as well. The other person may also translate the guilt into anger, and a defend-attack situation develops.

There is an inherent experience of guilt in special love relationships. At some level we "know" that we are taking from someone else to make ourselves whole, while we have little to give in return. This suppressed "knowing" is associated with repressed guilt. It builds up to such an extent that at some point the mere presence of the special person begins to remind us of what we are doing. As the guilt rises into the superficial subconscious, it is translated into anger. Then the individual, apparently for no reason, becomes irritated at his or her companion. He unconsciously picks a reason for his irritation—the way she cuts her hair, the type of clothes she wears or the way she talks. He may try to control this impulse, but ultimately the energy builds up and expression is demanded. A gentleman I know felt this irritation one day and held it in for as long as he could, but just as he and his wife were backing out of the driveway to go to a party, he could no longer contain it and blurted out, "Did you have to wear that dress?" Already feeling insecure, his wife was devastated, and she became defensive and angry. A mutual defend-attack scenario ensued. The emotional energy of repeated incidents such as that can build up until a full-blown special hate relationship results, with each blaming the other.

Even if the above-mentioned factors could be successfully repressed and the facade could be maintained to match the ego ideal, it still would not work. We would be left with a feeling of emptiness. Substitutions simply do not work. They are empty and devoid of the life-giving love and joy we really seek. The resultant boredom with our partner is the subtle depression caused by the first whiff of repressed fear and guilt coming to the surface. But as I have stated, behind this cloud of negative emotion lies the energy of love and joy we really want.

Following are some personal experiences that contributed to my understanding of the female-male special love relationship. Once while I was in meditation, a beautiful women appeared in a vision. I was sensually attracted to her. She said to me, "I am your Higher Self." I didn't then understand the meaning of the experience. Later I had a similar meditative vision, but this time the woman was not sensuous but seemed to be a wise teacher from whom I felt overwhelming, nurturing love. She said to me, "I am your Higher Self." Then came a message in which I was told that I was missing this nurturing feminine aspect of myself which I could only experience from within. Yet without realizing it I had been seeking it outside of myself, and in so doing I unconsciously attracted women to play supportive roles in my life, including the work place. But because I was coming from a perception of lack, I attracted women who were also lacking and who, therefore, were unable to provide either the support I wanted or the success I wanted at work.

These visions gave me insight into other experiences. I remembered that as a child, up until about three years of age, I wanted more than anything else to be a girl. I played with dolls and tried to stretch my pull-over shirts into dresses. Now I understood that by attempting to make myself into a girl, I was trying to experience the feminine aspect of myself from which I felt separated.

Shortly after the age of three, I translated my desire to be a girl into a desire to have a girl. I became attracted to the opposite sex. Most men love to be in that feminine energy, whether in the role of lover or son or brother. In the lover relationship, men are attracted to the female body, particularly the parts that most symbolize the feminine. Feminine energy is like a divine nectar to men. However, all the women in the world aren't able to satisfy that longing. Yet some keep trying to find it there. What men really miss is the feminine aspect of themselves.

Women, of course, have similar experiences from the feminine perspective, desiring to be in that strong, supportive masculine energy.

I chose to share this insight with a spiritual group in which I was participating. On the night the sharing was to take place a transvestite showed up in full drag. I had never seen him before nor have I seen him since. But he heard the story. In his willingness, the synchronicities of life brought him together with the information that would help him understand his unsatisfied and unsatisfiable urges.

For a variety of reasons, we make a number of different types of choices in attempting to find what we miss from sources outside ourselves. In our culture, a man seeking the feminine from a woman is considered better integrated than one seeking it by becoming a woman. Of course, the same holds true for women. Both methods lead to frustration. Resolution can only be found in the inner experience of the energy of the Higher Self. Once that energy connection is activated, the feminine and masculine energies will be expressed in a balanced way appropriate for one's cultural situation. This will bring to our relationships an experience of wholeness.

Does the solution to the problems of special love relationships lie in not having them? Should we avoid others because of their secret selves and facade patterns and wait until our own pattern is completely healed? No! We do need these relationships, not as substitutes for reality but to help us get in touch with reality. It is through these special relationships—in their disappointments—that we first get in touch with the secret self. As our hidden patterns repeat themselves in our relationships, we become better able to identify them so that we can begin to heal them. As we reach for the Higher Self in our relationships, they will teach us what the true experience of love is like. If we apply the healing formula, our relationships will serve that higher purpose and become experiences of joy.

It takes only one member of the relationship to transform it if the other has even a little bit of willingness. Here, intercessory prayer is an important tool. The other person doesn't consciously need to know the focus and intent of the more enlightened member of the couple. However, free will operates, and there will be a few who won't choose to change. Their fear may be too great for the moment. Detachment from outcome is important to allow the relationship to be redefined, and if appropriate, to allow the partners to go their separate ways. It may be best not to keep commitments made in the absence of wisdom. Our happiness does not depend on a relationship, although it will increase if shared within one. There are many different types of relationships in our culture in which this happiness can be shared.

Remember that what we miss and seek, in all our relationships, is our whole self, or our Higher Self, and through it, God.

For more readings on special relationships, see *A Course In Miracles* (T-15.V, VII; T-16. IV-VII; T-17.IV; T-18.I, II, V, VII).[17]

Chapter 11
FACADE PATTERNS

The secret-self and facade-self combination takes many forms, which are based on early life experiences and which result in certain predictable and repetitive patterns of behavior. Listed below are some patterns I have observed. These patterns may contain some components of the ego ideal but to a great extent are actually an out-picturing of the secret self. Although they may be obvious to others, they are usually not apparent to the individual who is attempting to maintain them.

Some Facade Patterns

- Attach and suckle
- Clasp and nurse
- Fix and control
- Use and lose
- Conquer and discard
- Conquer and possess
- Struggle and persevere
- Run and hide

These descriptive titles need little explanation except for the last one, so my comments about them will be brief. These patterns are discussed to help us recognize when we have been hooked as a perpetrator or as a victim so that we can focus on release. They are not intended to create a milieu of judgment. We all have participated in these patterns in one way or another, and yet we all are innocent. If we are involved with someone who exhibits one of these patterns, recognition of it may help us to depersonalize (detach from) the experience and allow us to be understanding and helpful to the one in need of love.

The attach-and-suckle individual has had enough positive exposure in early childhood to have hope that there is a source of nurturing in the world. However, he has not had enough nurturing to afford him satisfaction. In most cases, the hunger dates back to a perception of rejection that was initiated in the first year or so of life. At this age, the child's major source of nurturing is the mother. His or her primary sensory contact with the world is through oral contact, and the major source of physical nurturing is through the mother's nipple or a bottle held in her hand. If for some reason emotional nurturing through physical contact is prematurely disrupted, feelings of loss (grief) and rejection (guilt and fear) may be sown in the subconscious. This rejection experience may be real or imagined. Its effect is the development of an ongoing tendency to be in need of nurturing and to fear its absence. The individual will exhibit traits of neediness by clinging and demanding attention. An atmosphere of desperation pervades his or her behavior and tends to frighten people away. The clinging neediness may at first be flattering, but ultimately it becomes very draining. This individual will be frustrated not only because his behavior tends to put people off, but also because the unconscious energy of rejection pushes people away or attracts people who have a need to reject. This type of individual comforts himself with oral stimulation as if he were arrested in that early childhood period of oral interface with the environment. Such individuals have a tendency to keep their hands around their face and mouth. In psychological terminology, this individual exhibits an oral character structure.

The clasp-and-nurse individual has been programmed to define self as worthy by nurturing others, usually to the point of exclusion of self. He or she feels responsible for everyone else's happiness and success. This program, which has usually been modeled by significant individuals in the person's childhood, has become part of the ego ideal. The result is a "super mother," the object of whose mothering may be a person, group or organization. He or she may couple with an attach-and-suckle type or mold his or her partner into that role. It is, of course, impossible to make others happy. The attempt to do so inevitably fails, resulting in increasing fear and guilt, which are compounded by the repressed resentment arising from the self-sacrifice required to play this role. The pressure of this situation ultimately takes its toll.

The fix-and-control individual is similar to the clasp-and-nurse individual but may have a less benevolent and less overtly nurturing demeanor; he may be subtle and disarming or overtly guilt-inducing, whichever is required by the demands of his ego ideal. He may not need others to be happy but needs to control them so they will fit into his ego ideal. Also, controlling someone else helps to ease a sense of helplessness, temporarily repressing fear and guilt.

The use-and-lose individual needs someone to contribute certain elements to the ego ideal, but his or her interest in and commitment to the other person is not great. The need to control the other is temporary and limited to the short term. This type does not want the obligation of a long-term commitment because of the potential of losing independence and control. This pattern may be exhibited in individual or group relationships.

An example of the latter is an individual in charge of an organization with a stated goal and a list of planned projects required to meet that goal. Thus there is a legitimate reason for having a permanent, stable organization. Volunteers who share the vision and are able to contribute monetary support are enlisted. Meetings are held, funds are raised and projects are completed, but the leader of the organization remains in control of all aspects. Because duties are not appropriately delegated, talents are wasted. Volunteers and workers feel restricted, become discouraged and fall away from the organization. Another set of workers and volunteers is enlisted, more meetings are held, additional funds are raised and another project is completed. But, again, the restricting control of the leader becomes unbearable and those involved become discouraged and fall away. If the ego dynamic of the person in question doesn't change, the cycle will continue until people and funds are exhausted, and the mission of the organization is never completely fulfilled. Then the use-and-lose individual may slip into blaming and complaining or moaning and groaning.

A person prone to conquer-and-discard behavior feels empowered by the sense of conquest. The fun is in the successful hunt. Once the conquest is made the thrill is gone. The trophy may be on the wall for a while, but ultimately it is relegated to the attic to make room for new ones. The flattery that comes with someone new and different being attracted to him may soothe the feelings of inadequacy for a while, but when the partner becomes familiar, the relationship is no longer fulfilling. This individual initially seems interested in making a commitment, but the commitment is only to the extent required for the conquest, and eventually will be broken.

To the conquer-and-possess individual, ownership is almost as important as the conquest. Thus he has a keen interest in keeping the initial commitment but requires continued proof of his partner's steadfastness. This commitment doesn't mean that multiple objects for conquest and possession may not be desired and sought. Thus the conquer-and-possess individual may have both a wife and a mistress and would become very upset if either tried to leave or express independence.

Someone exhibiting the struggle-and-persevere pattern identifies himself by his ability to overcome obstacles, which he unconsciously attracts or consciously selects. The greater the struggle, the less guilt the individual is aware of, and the better he will feel about himself. However, after the goal is gained, emptiness and boredom surface. Another goal must be identified so the struggle and accomplishment can continue. True happiness, the real goal, is never obtained. You might recognize this person as a workaholic.

The individual with the run-and-hide pattern does not want to be here. Being here is too risky. It is as if he or she has been forced to go swimming but doesn't want to get wet. So he attempts to skim along the surface of life without getting too involved. Because he fears getting fully immersed in the world, but still needs a substitute reality by which to define himself, he becomes a dreamer and creates that reality in his imagination. The imagined reality may be close enough to the physical paradigm that it could be integrated into the physical experience if proper action were taken. However, to take action requires being here—to be engaged; thus the dreams seldom come to fruition. Ultimately the individual escapes into more dreams. Being involved in the details of everyday life and acting out these dreams are like diving into cold water, and that is too stressful.

This type of individual may have great difficulty making decisions, afraid that if he makes a wrong one he will experience dangerous consequences. Indecision and inaction or incomplete action is the usual pattern. He procrastinates, has a messy office and leaves a trail of mess behind him. He doesn't want to remain involved enough to clean up. It feels tedious, i.e. boring. The run-and-hide individual tends to watch too much television or spend an unbalanced amount of time reading fiction. These activities are escapes into alternative substitute realities, where there is no risk and where he finds refuge from those first feelings of depression. Such a person may be seen as all talk but no action. A temporary sense of satisfaction is felt in talk, which becomes a substitute for action.

The run-and-hide individual also tends to be emotionally aloof. To invest his emotions in this life is painful. He is right, actually, but he invests his emotions into an alternative dream and not reality. This is not detachment, for this individual is really attached to the physical world by virtue of his fear of it. In a state of denial, he exists in an alternative substitute reality that only he (and perhaps a few followers) experience. The degree to which this individual is able to relate to society is inversely related to the degree of fear he feels and the resultant need for withdrawal.

In addition to affording a sense of protection, withdrawal may also serve the need to passively-aggressively express anger and manipulate others to serve the ego needs.

A run-and-hide individual may have a schizoid character structure. This individual, under stress, may break down into full-blown schizophrenia.

I suspect that some cases of attention-deficit disorder are a result of the run-and-hide pattern. This disorder may manifest itself in quiet, out-of-touch daydreaming or, in the more active form, in disruptive behavior that may seem appropriate in the individual's fantasy world but not in the everyday world.

The run-and-hide pattern is usually established prior to birth. A person may have had an unpleasant experience in a previous life and a pleasant between-life experience that he is reluctant to leave; or he may have experienced strong rejection just before birth, resulting in fear and resistance to incarnation. Typically this resistance is evidenced by a significant delay in the onset of labor or prolonged, difficult labor. The run-and-hide individual is not infrequently delivered by Cesarean section. These birth difficulties do not produce the run-and-hide pattern but are products of it, since the consciousness of the incoming individual affects labor and delivery. Of course, the mother's fear can also negatively affect the birth process.

Because of their active imaginations, run-and-hide individuals tend to be visionaries. Not all dreamers and visionaries fall into the run-and-hide category, however. Being a dreamer or visionary is not necessarily a disadvantage; it can be a rather good trait if the individual is grounded and the dreaming is balanced with integrative action. If the run-and-hide dreamer has released enough fear, he may attract others to act on his visions, and in that way be associated with some success. If not, he will attract individuals who are also lacking, and thus failure will be assured.

More than one facade pattern may occur in any given individual, and they usually do. One pattern may be exhibited in one situation and another pattern in another situation. Usually one pattern will dominate. Also, incorporated into these patterns are the various styles of passive-aggressive and active-aggressive projection.

The emotional urgency that produces these patterns comes from repressed pain from the past. The patterns have been unconsciously created in an attempt to avoid this pain. Playing them out, however, does not solve the problem. Although they may seem to afford temporary relief, ultimately they will lead to more grief and frustration.

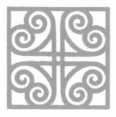

Chapter 12

THE EFFECT OF GUILT IN OUR CULTURE

Throughout written history humankind has never been able to conquer guilt. Attempts at disguise and repression have always failed. The final futile approach has been to accept oneself as a sinner with the hope that retribution can be negotiated by the act of becoming a self-informant, thus resolving guilt. This approach resulted in the concept of sin, guilt and punishment. This concept was reinforced by the punishing experiences in life caused by repressed guilt. Man's inability to see the energetic connection between his emotions and his outer experience led to the perception that the calamities of life were God's punishment for sin. Consequently, man thought he had been kicked out of the Garden of Eden by God, when in fact he had been kicked out by his own ego. Professing guilt (a form of moaning and groaning) was an attempt to release guilt by suffering.

One of the effects of fear and guilt was the degeneration and failure of the body. Guilt, which is anger toward self, contains the intent to punish. The subconscious mind of man identified with the body and thus directed punishment toward self by attacking the body, resulting in disease and physical pain. In addition, guilt manifested catastrophic circumstances in the environment, such as floods, famine, pestilence and earthquakes, that were also punishing to the psyche and the body.

Repressed guilt (self-hatred) is in effect a repressed death-wish. This hidden dynamic of the ego was recognized by Freud.[31] Unhealed humankind is subconsciously suicidal. At one level, we hate ourselves enough to kill ourselves. At another level, we are afraid to face this repressed self-hatred for fear that once it is discovered we will destroy ourselves.

The experience of disease, accidents and death caused by this unconscious dynamic witnesses to their "reality," causing us to have faith in them. This faith becomes a dynamic force independent of the guilt that initially caused the experience, and also contributes to the manifestation of the experience. These combined forces affect the body's DNA (genetic) program, causing the shut-down of cellular and glandular functions at a dictated time. The Old Testament characters who are described as living hundreds of years actually did so. Humankind gradually degenerated to a life expectancy even shorter than the current average of approximately seventy-two years.

This sin/guilt/punishment concept has permeated all cultures throughout recorded human history and can be seen in all of man's institutions, particularly religions, where it took the form of giving up something, including personal comfort, to appease the gods. The perception that justice required punishment led to the practice of surrogate punishment such as animal sacrifice and, in some cases, human sacrifice in an attempt to avoid our own. This practice also provided a way to disguise and vent guilt as projected anger.

In the early Hebrew tradition, the high priest symbolically placed his hands on a goat in order to transfer to the animal the sins of the community. The goat was then sent out to the desert to die as a way of banishing the sins. (This is where the term scapegoat originated.) At the time of Jesus, animal sacrifice was still part of the Jewish tradition. The money-changers that Jesus cast out of the temple were selling animals for sacrifice (AqG 72:6).[23]

Similarly, during Passover it was the custom to release a prisoner and send him into the desert to die. This was the purpose of the release of Barabbas. As in the scapegoat tradition, he was to take on the sins of the community. Barabbas, of course, had no intention of going out to die. In fact, he had bribed the Pharisees for his release and escape (AqG 168:1-6).[23] In the Christian religion, in spite of Jesus's teachings to the contrary, many of his followers, including the founders of orthodox* Christianity, continued the sin/guilt/punishment concept. To the orthodox Christian, Jesus was seen as the sacrificial lamb, taking on the sins of mankind and being punished in its stead. All those who accepted Jesus as their surrogate would be forgiven and saved.

Yet in the parable of the prodigal son, as told by Jesus (Luke 15:11), the son was welcomed back as a full family member without having to do penance, and the older brother was not punished in his stead. There was only celebration for the return of the once-missing son. He had only to change his mind and express the desire to return home to be fully reinstated as a son and brother.

The Bible tells us that before the creation of Eve and the eating of the apple, a deep sleep fell over Adam. Nowhere does it say that he woke up. Thus, it could be argued that everything that happened after Adam fell asleep occurred in a dream: he dreamed he sinned, that he was guilty and that God expelled him from the Garden of Eden to a life of pain and struggle.

In orthodox Christianity, more emphasis was placed on the Crucifixion than on the Resurrection. The Resurrection demonstrated that in the forgiving energy of love, sacrifice is impossible. Even a destroyed body can be brought back to life by love. Fear has no lingering effects in love's presence.

---

* Orthodoxy is used here in reference to both the Roman and Byzantine Churches and their descendants, as opposed to early Gnostic Christianity and some other more contemporary non-dominant Christian groups.

Not all early Christians accepted the concepts of orthodoxy, but the orthodox view held sway, particularly after the Roman emperor Constantine embraced it.

A hierarchy of male bishops and priests was established. Women were not allowed to speak in church, perhaps because they were more intuitive and forgiving. Members were discouraged from reading the Bible and were not taught to seek a direct experience of God through meditation. Forgiveness, which was sometimes sold for money, was meted out by the priest with a requirement for penance at his discretion. This gave the church a great deal of control over the population. When Constantine embraced orthodox Christianity, he used it to control the population, since the Empire had begun to lose its military power as a source of control. This is not to say that this was a conscious conspiracy; it was most likely the result of subconscious ego urges.

Today's mainstream Christian denominations have their heritage in orthodoxy, and although some changes have been made, the basic concept of sin, guilt and punishment remains. I don't mean to imply that some people have not found the kingdom of the soul through orthodox Christianity, for indeed, many have. There are many great saints in the orthodox church. I remain an active member of the United Methodist Church, which has its origins in orthodoxy. Among the mainstream denominations are individual congregations that encourage the freedom to explore beyond official dogma. Some individuals and congregations have attained a level of love that allows them to intuitively reach beyond orthodox dogma in their interactions with each other and with other faiths, while still maintaining conscious acceptance of orthodox dogma. They are willing to love without judgment. For the masses, however, orthodoxy has had a less than optimal influence because of its misleading beliefs.

As recorded in the New Testament, in the Gospel of John, Jesus said to the disciples, "I have much more to say to you, more than you can now bear [understand]. But when he, the Spirit of truth, comes, he will guide you into all truth" (John 16:12). And again, "Though I have been speaking figuratively, a time is coming when I will no longer use this kind of language but will tell you plainly about my Father" (John 16:25).

It was only after the discovery of the existence of the unconscious aspect of the mind and its collective nature, the analysis of the ego and the development of the concepts of modern physics that we were able to more fully understand what Jesus was saying. It is interesting timing that in 1975, the same year one outstanding source of this "plain talk," *A Course in Miracles*, was published, the Gnostic Gospels[73,95] were first translated into English. These early Christian writings had been discovered in a cave in the Nag Hammadi cliffs of Egypt in 1945. They were apparently hidden there when the Gnostic Christian movement was crushed after Constantine embraced orthodoxy. These writings indicate that the Gnostic Christians understood the teachings of Jesus more clearly than their orthodox counterparts.

In light of these recently revealed sources, it is much easier to go back to the Bible, which contains the writings approved by the orthodox church, and find truth—for it can indeed be found there if one is open to the intuitive wisdom of love. In Matthew 13:11-17, Jesus explains to the disciples why he spoke in parables: "Whoever has will be given more, . . . Whoever does not have, even what he has will be taken from him. . . . For this people's heart has become calloused; they hardly hear with their ears, and they have closed their eyes. Otherwise they might see with their eyes, hear with their ears, understand with their hearts." In other words, those who have love in their hearts will understand and gain. Those with anger in their hearts will misunderstand and lose. The ego has always misinterpreted the mystical teachings of the great masters and projected its own anger, specialness and greed into them. The key to understanding the Bible or any teaching is to approach it with the willingness to love—with love as the golden standard—letting go of the ego's need for specialness. Then, intuitive understanding will not be blocked.

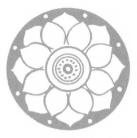

Chapter 13

MORE ON FORGIVENESS

In the beginning of the last chapter I referred to the attempt to conquer guilt. As long as we see guilt as real and something to conquer, the struggle will continue. We must become willing to be aware of the presence of guilt without struggling against it. Struggling makes it worse and results in more projection, substitution and suffering. We must simply allow love to replace it. Then guilt will be transcended without struggle. It will be lifted away through our willingness to focus on love and loving thoughts. The same is true of fear, anger and grief. (I realize that to replace "conquer" with "transcend" may seem like a play on words, but it is with words that we communicate, so their careful use may be helpful.)

To go back and undo a wrong or require the same of someone else so that we won't feel guilty or angry is to make the sin real and the guilt or anger justified. If we are willing to be free of guilt or anger without doing anything or requiring anything, love will simply lift it away. If we feel an urge to do something now to right a past wrong, it would be wise to examine our motives before acting. When our actions are motivated by love they are harmless and helpful. When they are motivated by guilt they are likely to be unwise and induce more unhappiness. We will be happier if we do not to try to conquer by action, but instead allow transcendence to occur. Then action, if appropriate, will be guided by the wisdom of love. Sometimes because we have difficulty forgiving ourselves, love will guide us to some act of undoing the past, not because it is required, but because we need that act to help let go of guilt. Love will guide us in that act of undoing without increasing fear.

In the blending of Eastern and Western cultures the word karma has become part of the daily language of many. To avoid confusion, some discussion of its meaning and its relationship to forgiveness is appropriate. Karma refers to the concept that current experiences are caused by past (ancient or recent) deeds. What you give is what you receive. This is an accurate depiction of the dynamics of consciousness and our world experience. The cycle of negative karma is interrupted by forgiveness. When we come to terms with repressed or conscious guilt from past misthoughts and deeds and forgive ourselves, karma is erased. If there is no memory or conscious recognition of the negative nature of past misthoughts or actions, the repressed guilt associated with them will attract to us a negative experience. As we embrace the negative emotions that surface, allowing them to be healed, and forgive as the impending situation starts to evolve, the threat dissolves and karma is gone. Once we have made a commitment to love, the power and wisdom of love will lead us to discover and release negative emotions in gentle and less frightening ways. For example, I have gotten in touch with a lot of repressed feelings in dreams, which lead to release and healing, thus avoiding the attraction of a negative experience in physical life. Following the formula on a regular basis heals repressed emotions and releases much karma before it can manifest in the physical experience. Yet, as I have said, if we seem to be threatened by an impending negative situation, it can be transmuted immediately through prayer and forgiveness.

This does not mean that every threat that seems to raise its head in our direction is necessarily attracted to us by our own negative energy. As I have said, the ego may project onto the "innocent." In such cases, if we are not vigilant, we may succumb to an instant, new karmic experience because we come to believe in the new threat, failing to remember that we are invulnerable when we choose to love, and then forget to forgive and see the potential perpetrator as innocent.

Forgiveness always involves letting go of the past and future. The past includes the past millisecond or something that occurred years ago. The only reality the past has is that which we give it in our minds. If we hold onto the past as a present reality, we will expect and have to guard against a future that reflects that past. In the process, we condemn the future, which tends to unfold as we expected. The only moment that exists is now. The past is not now. The future is not now. True love and happiness is always a **now** experience. If we depend on the past to change or the future to unfold in a certain way before we open to love, we will never find it. Then we will continue in the disappointments of false love, projection and suffering.

Someone may be standing before us threatening us right "now," or so it seems. Yet by the time the photons and sound reach our eyes and ears, causing nerve impulses, and by the time these impulses travel to the brain and create energy patterns that we interpret as seeing and hearing so that we become aware of the event, the event is already past—a fraction of a second ago. The body's experience is always a past-future experience. The future experience is shaped by our interpretation of the past experience, yet by the time the future arrives, it is already past.

Thus forgiveness may require us to let go of what seems to be happening in the present. If we are willing to do this, the next moment will be a manifestation of the peace we are willing to experience now. The threat will not be carried out against us. Because we choose not to perceive it or react to it emotionally, it will not become part of our reality. As we let all our concerns about the past and future go and focus on love and happiness, the love that is already in us will be given permission to express itself through our energy field, making our next moments a reflection of the peace we are willing to experience now

When we see our neighbors as innocent, we offer them that vision, and most will accept it. The gift of forgiveness becomes an effective force for change in the lives of others. This happens in the dynamics of the unconscious, and results in conscious behavioral changes. Those who do not choose to accept the love thus offered will become impotent in their attempt to affect us as long as we remain focused.

There are many symptoms that can tell us that forgiveness has not occurred—for example, a sudden urge to resist or judge when someone says or does something we consider outrageous. If someone makes an outrageous request of us, the tendency is to rise up in resistance. The request is made because that person feels his happiness and safety depends on it being honored. We rise up in resistance because we feel our happiness and safety depends on it not being honored, which is equally outrageous. Only the outrageous can define the outrageous. Our resistance makes the error seem real to both. The truth is, it doesn't matter. As a general rule, it is happier to forgive the outrageous and honor it, unless doing so will cause someone harm (ACIM T-12. 111.1-4).[17] The wise decision on what to do or not do will come from the peace that lies beyond the ego once the ego's fear and resistance are laid aside. This approach corresponds to the teachings of Jesus: "If someone wants to sue you and take your tunic, let him have your cloak as well. If someone forces you to go one mile, go with him two miles" (Matthew 5:40-41).

The outrageous thing may be something other than a specific request. It could be a practice or custom, or the specific terminology of an organization, institution or subculture that in our experience has been associated with a negative attitude or prejudice. It is important to take heed of our feelings of outrage and focus on forgiveness, for what we have not forgiven will be drawn to us by our negative emotional attachment until forgiveness is complete. There are no foolish requests or practices. There are only calls for love. As *A Course in Miracles* teaches, there are only two expressions on the planet: an expression of love and a call for love (ACIM T-12.I-3).[17] The happy response to either is love.

Chapter 14

THE BODY
AS A SYMBOL

I have described how the events of our lives are manifestations of our mostly unconscious emotional energy. As such, these events are like symbols in a dream, which, if we pay attention, will yield much information to facilitate healing and allow the dream to change.

The body, also a manifestation of this emotional energy, can also be thought of as a symbol of consciousness. All bodies are manifest in a characteristic way by the life force flowing through primary and secondary energy centers.[55] The energy of this life force is also the energy of our consciousness. In its unaltered state, in its normal quality, this energy is experienced emotionally as love, peace, joy, gratitude—all emotions that encompass the experience of love. Energy in the frequency of love manifests a perfectly functioning body, from its energetic interactions to its molecular and cellular experience. As discussed in Chapter 5, alterations of that energy, which is experienced as fear and the related emotions—guilt, anger and depression—may cause negative alterations in the molecular and cellular experience of the body.

Specific mental (perceptual) and emotional functions or issues affect the body's experience in characteristic ways. Thus, the body is an archetypal symbol.

The energy that forms the body is expressed through seven major energy centers and twenty secondary centers. The existence of these centers is recorded in mystical writings of Asia and the Middle East (the Eastern Vedas and the Jewish Kabala).[48] In Sanskrit, the language of the Vedas, the energy centers are called chakras, meaning wheels, referring to their wheel-like shape. Western technology now has confirmed the existence of energy points in the body as measured by variations in electrical potential.[6]

The chakras are traditionally numbered one through seven. The first major chakra is centered in the area of the coccyx. The parts of the body that are manifest from the energy of the first chakra include the coccyx; the lower sacrum; the anus, anal canal and rectum; and the nerves, muscles, soft tissues in this area. The kidneys and portions of the adrenal glands are also manifest from this energy center. Secondary first-chakra centers exist in the areas of the hands and feet and govern those parts of the body as well. The mental and emotional issues related to the first chakra have to do with material security in the physical plane. Fear, anger, guilt or depression related to financial security and other material issues may result in disturbance in any of these anatomical areas. The disturbance could appear as symptoms without obvious disease, as a disease with obvious molecular change or as an accident resulting in injury to these areas.

The second chakra is centered in the lower abdomen and pelvis. Tissues manifested by its energy include the external genitalia and internal sex organs, the lower lumbar and upper sacral vertebrae (centered in the area of the fifth lumbar and first sacral vertebrae), the lower abdominal wall, and the nerves, soft tissues, muscle and skin in these areas. Secondary centers are located in the wrist and ankles and include the heels and anterior lower legs. The mental and emotional issues related to this chakra have to do with the experience of pleasure, sexuality and creativity; they include one's relationship with a spouse, lover or potential lover, and in some cases with one's children. If there are negative emotions relative to these issues, pain or disease may develop in any of these areas.

The third chakra is centered in the solar plexus. A large energy center, it manifests the celiac nerve plexus in the upper abdomen, the pancreas, the liver and gallbladder, the spleen, the lower esophagus, the stomach, the small and large intestines, portions of the adrenal glands, the upper lumbar and lower dorsal vertebrae, and the muscles, soft tissues and skin in the mid back and upper abdomen. Secondary third chakras are centered in the areas of the forearms and calves. The mental and emotional issues related to this center have do to with control. This control has to do with all aspects of one's experience, but all control issues are ultimately related to personal identity. Negative emotions relative to this issue may manifest as abnormalities in any of the areas mentioned.

The fourth chakra is located in the area of the heart and thymus. Parts of the body produced by its energy include those organs as well as the alveoli of the lungs; the upper dorsal vertebrae, sternum and ribs; the breasts; and the nerves, muscles and skin in those areas. Secondary fourth chakras are in the areas of the elbows and the knees. The mental and emotional issues related to the fourth chakra include issues of the heart—that is, one's experience of love for a person or persons, a thing or a situation such as a job. If someone suffers a broken heart emotionally, he may physically experience a broken heart.

The fifth chakra is centered in the neck. The parts of the body manifested by its energy include the thyroid and parathyroid glands; the larynx, trachea and bronchi; the cervical vertebrae; the structures of the mouth, jaw and lower face; and the nerves, muscle, soft tissues and skin of the neck and mouth. Secondary fifth chakras are in the shoulders and hips, including the pelvic girdle. Its mental and emotional issues have to do with communication and expression. If someone has unresolved guilt over the way he has expressed himself or feels the need to communicate but will not because of fear, problems may develop in these areas. Asthma, for example, can be caused by repressed emotions.

The sixth and seventh chakras are closely related and will be discussed together. The sixth chakra is centered in the pituitary gland and the seventh in the pineal gland. Everything above the mouth and jaw is manifest from their energies. The mental and emotional issues related to these energy centers have to do with wisdom (how we see and interpret the world and ourselves in it) and spirituality (how we relate to our spiritual nature). There are no secondary sixth or seventh chakras.

Since the source of this information is mystical and these phenomena cannot be explained by molecular causes, the scientific community has not yet committed the resources needed for large-study statistical validation of these relationships. In the meantime, we will have to rely on individual case experiences—in other words, anecdotes. To deny the validity of these experiences out of hand, to withhold the information and to not collect more data that would lay a more "acceptable" scientific basis for validation is to delay the advancement of medical science and prevent people from experiencing better results from their medical therapies.

The cases that I will now relate are all true. Again, some of the non-essential, non-medical aspects, including names, have been altered for the sake of privacy.

A young woman, Susan, came to my office with a six-month history of fatigue, lethargy, somnolence, intermittent sore throat, swollen lymph nodes in the neck, morning nausea and vomiting and chronic pain between the shoulder blades. She had been seen by several doctors but had received no specific diagnosis. Her symptoms fell into the category of chronic fatigue syndrome, which is a diagnosis made after other classifiable diseases have been excluded.

When I questioned her about her mental/emotional experience

she came up with nothing. Her relationships were peaceful. She had no traumatic memories or financial stress. She did say her work was stressful but that she was able to put it in the back of her mind. That statement alerted me to pursue that area of her life. The only stress she was aware of concerned the tight schedule at work, but this didn't seem to me to be the issue. Finally I simply said to her, "Your heart is broken." That was all it took: she started to cry. It was like sticking a pin in a balloon filled with water. She sobbed uncontrollably for a while and finally, when she was more relaxed, was able to relate the real problem. She was a nurse and worked in a pediatric intensive care unit dealing with newborn infants, most of whom were premature. They had to be hooked up to IVs and tubes and seemed to suffer. Many of the infants died, in spite of all that was done. The emotional impact of this experience was compounded by the fact that as a young woman she expected to become a mother one day, so she saw the infants as potentially her own. She felt helpless, and her grief in this experience was so great that she repressed it. My saying, "broken heart," brought her grief to the surface. The reason I was drawn to her heart was the pain in her upper back, which is in the area of the fourth chakra. Her nausea, vomiting, and fatigue were related to her perception of a lack of control, a third chakra issue. Her repressed, unexpressed emotions involved the fifth chakra, which resulted in the sore throat and swollen cervical lymph nodes. The somnolence was an attempt to escape what she had not wanted to face.

First we approached the problem with cognitive therapy. I introduced her to some of the ideas in this book and gave her alternative ways to view her situation. I suggested that the infants were not as she saw them. They were not bodies but minds that had not yet completely committed to focusing themselves into the body. They were deciding whether to stay and restore health to the bodies they had inherited in their choice to incarnate, or to leave. If they found it too difficult, considering their possible limited abilities, they might abandon the effort.

I shared with her the experience of a friend of mine who could remember being a three and one-half pound premature infant with respiratory distress syndrome. Not yet able to relate to the world through her senses, she remembers hearing in her mind, in expanded awareness, the words, "If you want to stay, you have to breath." So she focused all her attention on breathing and survived.

As stated in Chapter 5, the mind predates the body. If a mind planning to come into this realm finds one body unsuitable, it will withdraw and wait for another one. Ultimately, it will select a body that will bring it into the proximity of the people it needs or wishes to relate to in its incarnation. If it needs to be in a particular family and the first body dies, it may become the next child the mother of that family has. If the mother has no more children, it may choose to incarnate as the child of a sister or someone close to the family so that it will have the opportunity to interact with whomever is most appropriate.

I also explained to Susan how she could use the energy of love accessed through prayer to help the infants. She could focus the healing energy of her love by intent and touch, and thus assist in healing the energy fields of the infants' bodies. This love would also help heal their fears about coming into the incarnation or about their ability to sustain life in the body. Even then, however, the infants-to-be might decide not to stay. Next we did some prayer and meditative work to heal the emotions with which she was now getting in touch. I gave her the formula described in Chapter 6. We scheduled another appointment in two weeks. No other therapy was prescribed.

Two weeks later she returned and reported that she had had no more symptoms after the initial visit. I saw her in a non-client setting about a year and a half later, and she was still symptom-free.

Barbara was in her mid-thirties. She had a two-year history of low-back and left-hip pain. Approximately six months previously she had undergone surgical removal of the greater trochanteric bursa of the left hip because of chronic bursitis. This gave her relief for only a week or so. She was obviously in pain, distraught and depressed. She had been worked up extensively and brought in her X-rays for review. They revealed accentuation of the lumbosacral angle, which produced increased strain on the lumbosacral ligaments that support the torso.

After briefing her about my approach, I explained the mental-emotional equivalents of her symptoms that were the energetic cause of her disease. Because of the pain in her left hip, I knew she had a communication problem. Because of the pain in her lower back (L5-S1), I knew she had emotional issues related to her experience of pleasure and/or her relationship with her husband. That the hip problem was on her left side also suggested it concerned her communication as a woman with a man. (The left side of the body seems to be an archetypical expression of the feminine aspect, and the right, the masculine aspect.)

With a little questioning, we soon discovered the root of the problem. She had grown up with a sense of responsibility for everyone else's pleasure to the sacrifice of her own. If others were unhappy, she felt guilty. Thus the fear associated with guilt drove her to go out of her way to see to the needs of others, particularly her husband. Because of the guilt, she didn't feel free to communicate her own needs. Her problem was a combination of second and fifth chakra issues. A symbolic way to view her body, specific for her situation, is that she was carrying the weight of the world on her shoulders, and it was breaking her back.

I shared with her new perceptions and a different way to see her situation, explaining that because we are all connected in the energy field of consciousness, what is for her highest good is also for the highest good of everyone else. I suggested that she approach her husband affirming trust and love, and a willingness to see those qualities in him. I taught her the formula, and we did some guided meditative work to release old belief systems and emotions. She was sent on her way, after having been scheduled to return in two weeks for a follow-up appointment.

At the appointed time of Barbara's return, the receptionist notified me that she had arrived. I glanced into the waiting room and saw a young woman, but it didn't seem to be my patient. When I asked the receptionist where Barbara was, she confirmed that the woman in the waiting room was indeed Barbara. I looked again and in amazement realized that this vibrant, attractive woman was the same person I had seen two weeks ago. The strain of worry and pain was no longer on her face. She was bright and cheery with sparkling, alive eyes. In our session she told me that the pain had left the day of her first visit. She had talked with her husband and was changing her life style. After further cognitive work, she was discharged.

Barbara remained totally free of pain for six months, at which time it returned. This recurrence resulted from the stress of new relationship problems with her husband. Aware of the connection of her pain to conscious or repressed emotions, she had tried to work on the problem herself but without success. However, she had delayed her return because she didn't want to admit failure. This raises another issue to which I have previously referred—the guilt that arises once one accepts responsibility for experiences that are less than perfect. The guilt is, of course, inappropriate, but it must be acknowledged and dealt with. This patient needed additional cognitive work to help her deal with the changes in her marriage.

We also revisited a childhood event that on first review had seemed innocuous but turned out to be a significant trauma in need of healing. As a very young child, Barbara's father was stationed overseas during the Korean conflict. She had unconsciously retained the pain associated with the perception that he had left because of her. In other words, she had inappropriately accepted responsibility for his leaving, causing repressed guilt. More meditative work was required to release the residue of negative emotions, and she did well.

Young children frequently think of themselves as the center of the reality that revolves around them and may feel responsible for what happens to others in it. This may carry over into adulthood. We can influence others, but since life is a collective, free-will experience, we do not individually cause the actions of others. Their own consciousness is cause.

At the other extreme is the fear that children have related to their sense of helplessness, or the loss of control over the world around them. The case of a young diabetic illustrates this point. In her pre-teen years, prior to the onset of her juvenile diabetes, Nancy's world seemed to fall apart. Her grandmother, to whom she was very attached, died; her older brother left home; and her older sister began to cause problems in the family. Nancy's perception was that she had no control over the events around her and thus was unable to be assured of her own safety and happiness. As a result of this third chakra issue, her pancreatic endocrine cells failed. She developed diabetes melitis. In her fear of loss of control, she symbolically lost the unconscious ability to control her metabolism. She took conscious control by learning to check her blood glucose and administer insulin.

She later married. When her husband was shipped overseas by the Army, for no apparent reason she went into a diabetic coma. Her husband was given a permanent charity furlough so he could be with his sick wife. As she recovered, she remembered thinking, "I can control the entire United States Army." This example illustrates the secondary gain of illness. Patients may unconsciously attempt to control events around them through their illnesses. This is actually manipulation by inducing guilt. In such cases, healing will not occur until belief in the need for the secondary gain is released. This is seldom a conscious dynamic, and getting the patient to face and release the need sometimes seems difficult.

Another example of manipulation through guilt for secondary gain is the case of Jane, who was chronically ill to the extent that she had to be constantly cared for and chauffeured by her husband. Her illness trapped him. Her repressed premise was: "He can't leave me because I am sick. He would feel too guilty." She neither trusted her husband to love her nor believed in her ability to be happy without him. So she unconsciously manifested the illness to ensure his presence.

A common and classic example of the third chakra issue of control is sea-sickness. The experience of movement is mediated not only by visual cues, but also through the vestibular apparatus of the inner ear. However it is not the stimulation of the vestibular apparatus that causes the nausea and vomiting. A person may not be consciously aware of fear while being tossed around in a boat, but the action stimulates unconscious fears related to control. The resultant symptoms are due to alteration of third chakra energies. The threshold for these symptoms varies from individual to individual, depending on unconscious programming. Place the individual behind the wheel of the boat where he may have a sense of being in control, and sea-sickness is less likely to occur. Sometimes stimulating the third chakra directly or focusing attention on it may prevent the symptoms—thus explaining home remedies that involve placing something over the abdomen. One such remedy calls for placing an aspirin in the navel. I have actually seen this work.

Moving back to the second chakra, Mary, a married women in her late thirties, came to me complaining about two years of chronic vaginitis, which had been unresponsive to therapy. Unless you have had this condition it may not seem like a significant problem, but imagine two years of itching and irritation in an area of the body on which we place so much emotional significance. It didn't take long to discover that she was also suffering from chronic irritation with her husband. With some perceptional work, prayer and meditation, she was able to release her annoyance with him, and her vaginitis cleared up and never returned. Mary's change in attitude also affected her husband, who changed his behavior; as a result, there was less temptation for her to be irritated.

The seriousness of the physical problems or life situations we experience reflects the intensity of the emotional energy involved. I had the opportunity to work with a young woman who had been treated for carcinoma of the cervix. Elizabeth had been married to an abusive husband, and the marriage had ended in a bitter divorce prior to the onset of the cancer. The cancer seemed to be in remission after surgery and radiation therapy, but she continued to be troubled by persistent back pain. Her cancer and now her persistent pain were a manifestation of her extreme anger. Not only was she still feeling rage toward her ex-husband, who was still threatening her, but she was also distressed over a relationship with another man who had promised a long-term commitment leading to marriage, but kept yo-yoing between her and his wife.

Initially during therapy Elizabeth showed symptomatic improvement. But when her boyfriend returned to his wife, her pain became so severe that she required hospitalization. Repeat diagnostic studies revealed recurrent carcinoma. As we worked on the emotional equivalents of her problem, she remembered thinking, "If I get sick, that will really show him." Her anger had motivated a desire to make her boyfriend feel guilty for leaving, so she got sick. Consciously it was just an "idle thought." She would not have consciously chosen to suffer pain just to get back at him. Yet what seemed like a transient, harmless thought actually represented the tip of an iceberg—the iceberg representing a lot of repressed emotional energy. Now she found herself facing a difficult situation. She had to deal not only with anger toward the men in her life, but also with the fear of a potentially fatal disease.

It is actually not any harder to heal cancer than vaginitis or bursitis. But because of the strong collective faith we have in cancer and the intensity of the negative emotions and perceptions associated with certain types of cancers, it is often difficult to experience healing. For most people, to do so requires a great deal of discipline, but it can be and is done. Changing the mind and reprogramming the subconscious seem like difficult tasks. Thus the paradox: it is not hard, but it is, because we make it so. (In the experience of a false reality which is turned inside out or upside down, all truths are paradoxical.)

Men, of course, also have second chakra problems, including soft tissue irritations, infections, hyperplasia, benign neoplasms and malignant neoplasia. Prostatic hyperplasia and prostatic carcinomas are common. A less common problem is carcinoma of the testis. A young man came to me with a malignant tumor of the testicle. As we searched for the source of second chakra stress, initially everything looked positive. About three months prior to the discovery of the tumor Paul had become engaged. Even change that we think of as positive can be stressful because all change involves unknowns, and there lingers in our collective consciousness a fear of the unknown. However, in this young man's case, there was a deeper problem. He had dated his fiancee several years previously, but she had left him for another man. Now that they were back together and about to get married, his jealousy and anger began to resurface. As these emotions built up, he was unable to resolve them; as a result they caused an alteration in second chakra energy leading to the DNA mistake that resulted in the tumor. Through willingness, prayer and meditative work, he experienced emotional healing. He experienced physical healing through removal of the testicle. He married and went on with his life.

A first chakra problem was being experienced by another young man who, while employed, was looking for a job elsewhere. Jake feared that his current employer would find out and fire him. As he perceived it, his security was threatened. His fear manifested in his left foot, not a serious problem but a painful one. The body in this case had become a symbol of the dynamics of his situation: as he was stepping forward with the right foot while being supported by the left, he was afraid that something would happen to that support—the rug might be pulled out from under his supporting left foot. This was not a difficult problem to resolve, once the dynamics were pointed out and the appropriate prayer, meditation, affirmations and focus were instituted.

Ear and eye problems may be related to being disturbed by what one hears or sees. Chronic ear problems in children, in my experience, are almost always caused by conflicts in the family. Young children are very susceptible to the emotional energies of those close to them. Thus, the most rapid success in treating children comes in examining and dealing with family dynamics.

In working with pre-verbal children, intuitive work is necessary. Since our minds are not separate this can be done with willingness, openness and trust in the process. In the case of one young child, while assisting another practitioner, I blended my consciousness with the child's, felt her pain and understood the issues with which she was dealing. She had developed illness and almost died. She recovered from the illness but failed to thrive and develop normally because of her unresolved fear. The fear was related to conflict between her mother and father, and a threatened divorce. During the period of illness, as she lay in a coma, the child contemplated whether to stay or leave. The effect of her illness was to bring the family back together. In her expanded consciousness she recognized the willingness of the parents to change and decided to stay. However, her commitment to stay was guarded. After we worked with the child and her parents spiritually, her fears began to resolve, and she improved remarkably.

Parents, you are not guilty if you have a sick child. Remember, you are innocent, doing the best you can, and so is the child. There are many different energy dynamics operating in the illness of children other than the ones I have described. Children have their own mental-emotional problems to contend with and their own subconscious minds to heal, and usually they are born with pre-existing negative emotional dynamics that cause them to be attracted to certain situations and that influence their reaction to those situations.

A child may be born specifically to experience the unconditional love of its mother to heal an old pain. Once this is accomplished, the child may, at an expanded level of consciousness, choose to die, perhaps of sudden infant death syndrome. Is it loving to leave grieving parents? Perhaps the parents had a great deal of repressed grief from a past event that still needed healing. The death of the child would bring all their repressed grief to the surface, giving them the opportunity to face it and heal it. Prior to incarnation the child was at some level aware of these dynamics, which determined its choice to incarnate into that particular family. Thus the highest good of all was served.

The highest good is most immediately and easily facilitated if the individual mind turns the choice of incarnation over to the higher wisdom of love. Because of fear and resultant attachments, some incarnations do not occur under the guidance of higher wisdom. Free will operates to some extent in this area of choosing as well. However, at any time the choice can be made to turn to love so that the effects of a past poor choice will be transcended. Every experience is an opportunity, so in this sense, there are no poor choices.

The next two cases illustrate problems with the sixth and seventh chakras. One involves an intelligent, well-educated man who was intellectually arrogant and often disparaging of those not as educated. The "poetic justice" of his experience was his senile dementia, which led to the failure of his intellect and the inability to use his education. His unrecognized repressed guilt of judgment was the administrator of the "poetic justice," not God.

In the other case, a man was afraid to utilize his intellect. As an accountant, his fear was experienced as pressure related to the volume of work to be done under certain time constraints and the possibility of making mistakes. Unaware of other ways of seeing and handling the situation, he had the conscious thought, "I'm tired of thinking." As he got older, he too developed senile dementia and lost the ability to think. His wife acknowledged that he seemed happier and less irritable; however, she made all his decisions, even to the point of dressing him.

These are just two examples of the mental and emotional equivalents of senility; there are many more, and each case is unique. A particular disease will have a predictable molecular and anatomical expression from individual to individual, but may have quite varied mental and emotional equivalents. The solution and prevention for all are found through use of the formula.

I will share with you a personal experience of my own to illustrate a fifth chakra problem and how healing may be associated with external experiences that can cause shifts in perception. One of my recreational activities used to be TV channel-surfing. One day I happened to flip to a religious channel televising a young Pentecostal evangelist who was speaking at a local church. His performance was loud and boisterous with a lot of jumping and prancing. I thought what I saw was ridiculous, but I kept watching so I could laugh with ridicule at the spectacle. The church had a regular time slot, and I returned to it several times over the next few weeks so I could have a good laugh and "enjoy" the feeling of ridicule. I subsequently had a dream that I later understood represented two aspects of me: a foreman (my judgment) who was drunk and out of control; and a hard-working, sober laborer (my experience) with a cast covering his jaw. The next day I came down with the worst toothache I had ever had. I made an emergency trip to the dentist, who told me I needed a root canal. He was willing to do it that day, but I was scheduled to fly out of town that afternoon for the weekend, and the dentist could not guarantee that I would make the flight if he operated. So I elected to take some pain pills and see if I could make it through until Monday.

I managed. Monday morning I went to work anticipating that I would call the dentist and have the dental work done. But something intervened. An employee who happened to be Jewish, not knowing of my dental affliction or my TV ventures into ridicule, showed me a newspaper ad featuring the evangelist. He was going to speak at the same local church, and the ad was promoting the evangelist's ability to perform dental miracles. This synchronicity was too great to ignore. I knew I had to "eat crow" and attend his service.

Anne, my wife-to-be, attended with me. We sat in the back so we could make a quick exit if we became too uncomfortable. In his sermon the evangelist alluded to those who sat in the back because of their fears. But as I listened to him speak, I realized that he was speaking the truth and from the heart and that most of those in attendance were sincere in their love and enthusiasm. Their behavior of dancing and shaking to the music was an expression of that enthusiasm. In the past I had gone through similar gyrations and noise-making at rock-and-roll dances and thought nothing of it. I had watched Mick Jaggar of the Rolling Stones perform and had been entertained. In fact, the minister's style of delivery was similar to Jaggar's, and I realized that it was entertaining and that it kept my and the congregation's attention focused. I realized I was simply witnessing a cultural difference and let go of my judgment that a religious service had to entail sitting quietly in the pew while a minister delivered a calm, somewhat intellectual sermon. Interestingly, in his sermon the evangelist referred to the ridicule King David got for dancing before the Lord (2 Samuel 6:12-23). I realized this minister was no fool. I no longer felt the emotional energy of ridicule. At the end of the service, the evangelist asked those who had dental problems to have someone next to them place his or her hand on their jaw as he prayed and to accept healing. Anne placed her hand on my jaw, and my pain resolved and I did not have the root canal.

The repressed guilt associated with judging my brother, the evangelist, as a fool produced the "appropriate" retribution: the toothache. To my subconscious, the thought was as real as speaking the words. Once I realized I was in error, I let go of my judgment, forgave the evangelist for being different and forgave myself. I was then open to receive the unaltered healing energy of love that is always immediately available when we are willing. It is important to note that I was never consciously aware of the feeling of guilt. The guilt was hidden in the physical pain in my mouth. In my willingness, the events around me led to an experience that brought to me the appropriate understanding so that I could release the hidden guilt.

As I have indicated, the body is not only an archetypical symbol, it can also symbolize the unique circumstances of an individual's consciousness. I had the opportunity to work with Dianne, who had bronchogenic carcinoma with metastasis. When she was a child, her mother had been cold and distant, and wouldn't allow her to express her feelings, particularly feelings of love. Not surprisingly she had asthma as a child. Now as an adult she was still unsuccessfully attempting to smother her emotions. One of the major symptoms of her pulmonary tumor was a sensation of smothering.

Dianne was consciously aware of feeling guilty. The guilt was worse than the physical pain of her disease. She had been very close to her father, and on his death-bed he had made her promise never to place her mother in a nursing home. When her mother became senile, fell and fractured her hip, Dianne seemed to have no choice but to put her in a home. She felt guilty not only for breaking the promise to her father but also for her anger toward her mother. She was also experiencing some mental confusion due to the spread of the tumor to the brain, symptoms not unlike those of her mother's senility. But most of the physical pain was in the right hip. It was the right hip that her mother had fractured.

This case offers an example of a commitment that was not made in wisdom. As I have discussed earlier, commitments made in the absence of wisdom are not necessarily meant to be kept. Nor are they necessarily meant to be broken. We can change our decisions or change the circumstances the decision produced. Any decision, including one to keep or break an old commitment, is best made based on wisdom that comes from a peace from within, independent of external circumstances.

In another case, a woman in her early thirties came to see me because of food allergies. Her reactions to foods had become so severe and unpredictable that she was afraid to eat unless she was in the parking lot of an emergency room. She related to me that once she had been quite pretty but that her body had changed. She had lost too much weight and was now much too thin to be considered pretty by her own standards. Furthermore, as an African-American it had been her perception that the relatively light tone of her skin was a feature of her beauty, but inexplicably she had become quite dark.

She was married to an emotionally abusive man who was failing to come home at night. She suspected he was involved with another woman. In the past she had experienced pain and stress, a lot of it in the form of sexual harassment, at the hands of men who were attracted to her because of her beauty. But worse in her view were the attacks from women jealous of her good looks. She remembered wondering if it would be better to be ugly. On top of that, her husband's suspected philandering made her feel ugly. These perceptions and their emotional energy were producing for her, in part through food allergies, an ugly body.

We proceeded with intensive cognitive and supportive perceptual work, which included deprogramming her from a belief that she would be victimized if she were pretty while giving her a sense of her true identity so that she would be less vulnerable to the words and actions of others. I instructed her on the use of the formula. I also had her introduce new foods to her diet, one at a time. Within three weeks it was evident that she was on the road to recovery. She no longer had allergies, she was putting on weight, and to my amazement her skin color began to lighten. In addition, her husband started staying home and became more attentive after she began to focus on him mentally with the intent to forgive and love. This program, of course, required willingness to let go of the past and to see perfection in him as if that past had not occurred.

Depending upon an individual's unique experiences, he may develop a propensity for negative emotional energy to express through one particular chakra system over the others. Negative energy from one system may shift and affect another. Also, there is overlap among the systems in regard to areas of the body affected. The third chakra may also affect the thigh; the fourth chakra may affect the pelvis; and the fifth chakra may affect the torso.

Some diseases are systemic and not as easy to associate with a specific chakra system as when symptoms are more localized. However, the general nature of the presentation of the disease may lead to the mental equivalent. For example, fear related to loss of control may result in loss of control of the body as in multiple sclerosis. This has been my observation, as well as the observation of others.[51]

Individuals with breast cancer are generally over-nurturing types (clasp and nurse). They are the super-mothers of people or organizations.

The pressure and sacrifice involved in playing such a role or the perceived failure in playing that role are associated with fear, guilt and anger. The physical equivalent in this situation is that the breast is being sucked from the body. Less serious breast disease may occur when the emotional energy is less intense but the issues are similar.

Immune suppression and disturbance cause one to be susceptible to infections and prone to develop allergies or autoimmune disease. As I discussed earlier, the way the disease presents itself in the body and the effect it has on the individual's situation will be symbolic of the mental equivalents.

One patient I worked with had problems with hay fever. Other aspects of her life were going well. In analyzing her past, we discovered that in her early childhood she had been happy until the family had made a disruptive move. Adjustments were finally made and life seemed good again. Then her father became ill. As a result of these disruptive events, she developed the unconsciously programmed perception that whenever things went well something terrible would happen. One of her favorite activities as a child was visiting her grandmother's farm, where pollens were plentiful. To protect herself from another disaster she unconsciously developed allergies to the pollens. This prevented things from becoming too good. With cognitive therapy, prayer and meditation she was able to release the perception and the negative emotional energy related to the past. Her allergies cleared, and she was able to do without her allergy shots and antihistamines.

Finding something in the context of current experience may give a hint of the perception or emotional trauma that is at the root of the problem. John had been doing well until he reached the age of 44. Then his luck ran out. He lost one job after another, his health began to deteriorate, his vision failed and his prescribed glasses would not maintain correct vision for any length of time. As we examined his past he revealed that as an adolescent, to get the attention of his peers, he had been a rebellious trouble-maker. His mother, whom he caused a lot of pain, was 44 years old during the peak of the rebellion. When he reached that age, the repressed guilt began to surface and affect his life. Once he became aware of this guilt and its relationship to his current experience, we could deal with it perceptually and through prayer and meditation.

As I have indicated, emotional traumas long forgotten but not dealt with will leave vortexes of negative emotional energy that are self-perpetuating and added to by repeated negative events. These events take different forms, but they have the same perceptual and emotional content of the initial trauma. One example of this phenomenon is the experience of Evelyn, a woman in her mid thirties who came to me with a six-year history of severe pain in the posterior cervical and occipital areas. Approximately one year prior to her visit, an arteriogram had revealed a bulge in an intracranial artery in the proximity of the ninth, tenth and eleventh cranial nerves. Because of the possibility that the pain was caused by pressure of the artery on these nerves, a craniotomy (opening of the skull) had been performed in order to surgically relieve the suspected pressure. In addition, the eleventh nerve had been severed for pain relief. She had relief for about three months, then the pain returned.

During the period of our analytical work in search of the mental-emotional equivalent of her pain, she had a dream in which she saw a seven-year-old girl in a hospital gown who was lost and in need of help. While relating this dream in a deep, relaxed state, she remembered an event she had experienced when she was seven. She was watching a rabbit in a fenced pen when a dog jumped the fence and viciously attacked the rabbit. The dog bit into the back of the rabbit's neck and head, ripping away the tissues and killing it. The attack horrified her, but she managed to repress her feelings, then the memory. Later, however, as she began to experience stress in her adult life, the negative emotions began to out-picture as symptoms corresponding to that horrible experience. The pain Evelyn was now feeling was equivalent to having the back of her head and neck ripped out. Within the two-year period prior to the onset of her physical symptoms, she had gone through separation and divorce from a verbally abusive husband. It was as if life was attacking her just as the dog had attacked the rabbit, and emotionally she was feeling ripped apart. After a few weeks of perceptual therapy, meditative release and other types of negative energy-release and relaxation therapies, her symptoms were so improved that she no longer required medication.

How an individual out-pictures the effect of fear in the body depends to some extent on the thought energy of the family into which the individual is born. This thought energy affects the energy field of the body, and in some cases results in DNA, chromosomal, and tissue-antigen abnormalities. Thus we can predict certain probable outcomes based on family history and molecular and genetic studies. As I have stated, however, we are not ultimately limited by those markers. Our limitations are those we accept in consciousness.

In addition to familial negative energy, collective cultural negative energy may also manifest itself in disease. This energy is passed through the collective energy field of consciousness to become a collective or contagious experience. Some of these energies manifest in forms that can be identified, such as viruses, which may be passed from one individual to another. But remember, the collective physical experience is a manifestation of collective consciousness, which is contributed to by individual consciousness. Each individual unit of consciousness still has the freedom to transcend the effect of collective consciousness. Most people have variable susceptibility to these negative energies because of lack of vigilance and doubts. However, at any time with proper vigilance, we can exert our free will and allow negative effects to be healed.

A few years ago a flu epidemic was in full swing in Richmond. It had been going around the office, and one Friday afternoon, shortly after I got home, it suddenly hit me: high fever, shaking, chills and terrible malaise. All I felt like doing was giving in to it by going to bed and knocking myself out with medication in order to sleep through it. But I was scheduled to attend a conference the next morning. I mustered all the energy I could and focused on being well. I prayed, meditated and verbally affirmed my health and my connection with the healing love of God. I prayed until two in the morning, then allowed myself to fall asleep. When I woke up the next morning, I was totally well, without any residual symptoms. The epidemic had been a particularly severe strain of the influenza virus, debilitating people for about a week on the average. I cannot relate my succumbing to the virus to a particular chakra system. However, my immune system was not performing to perfection, and there had also been the thought energy that I might get the virus. In this case, the recovery occurred through an exercise of will, intense focus and a willingness to love and be loved.

I could share many other cases, but the point is adequately made with these few. I am not presenting this material as scientific proof of the premise I feel it supports. However, my own experience leaves me convinced of its validity and practicality. Herein lies the solution to the national health crisis. These cases are anecdotal, and trust in the observer is required, but they reveal enough to point to areas and approaches for further research. Skepticism is healthy if it is true skepticism—that is, an omni-directional or non-exclusive skepticism with an openness to any possible conclusion. However, studies must be designed that take into account the practitioner's faith in the therapeutic process, whatever process is being used, and the ability of the practitioner to share that belief with the patient. To separate the subjective experience of the practitioner from the healing process removes an essential ingredient. It removes the healer. The doctor who approaches a patient with no faith in what he is doing is not a healer and offers the patient very little. The true physician must have hope, faith in the process and, above all, love for the patient and himself.

Chapter 15

COOPERATING WITH THE MOLECULAR "REALITY" FOR HEALING AND HEALTH

One purpose of this book is to let it be more commonly known that we are not victims of the molecular world. Nor are we ultimately subject to its laws. These laws are manifestations of consciousness, not the cause of consciousness. Humankind was not made for the world; the world was made for humankind. To those centered in the ego, this is a statement of arrogance. To the enlightened, however, it is simply a statement of truth and an acknowledgment of responsibility. We are created to co-create. The Bible states that man was given dominion over the world (Genesis 1:26). In other words, man's consciousness has dominion over the world. Consciousness is cause, and the world is effect. If humankind were to be responsive to its true nature, this role would be a loving blessing, not the curse it has seemed to be throughout history.

The predictable, ongoing and dynamic interactions of the world of nature—physical, molecular and bio-molecular—are manifestations of the intent of consciousness. These interactions are powerful because consciousness is powerful. We can learn about them and use them for our benefit. At our present level of awareness, some of these physical and molecular events are perceived to be essential to our health and well-being. Although we are not limited by natural laws, until mastery of mind is complete, it is easier to align with and accept the good in them rather than to try to ignore and live counter to them.

The body at humankind's present level of evolvement has certain requirements: food, including vitamins, minerals and essential amino acids; water; air; and a certain range of ambient temperature. Adequate exercise and rest are also important. When the body becomes ill, medicine and surgery can be beneficial.

The immediate effect of surgery is quite obvious and predictable. For most people, it would be easier to have diseased tissue surgically removed when clinically appropriate than to attempt some alternative therapy. However, the long-term results, the degree of immediate or long-term pain and the presence or absence of complications will be determined by the patient's mental-emotional state. An unresolved mental-emotional equivalent may result in surgical complications, recurrence of the disease or the manifestation of another disease.

An example of a less-than-optimal surgical outcome is a woman with a clasp-and-nurse ego facade. She was the supermother to an unappreciative extended family. Not surprisingly, she developed breast cancer. The situation and the perceptual problem were not resolved prior to her mastectomy. The surgery was a cosmetic disaster with infection, scarring and disfigurement. The already negative aspect of her emotional state was heightened by the fact that prior to surgery her health insurance had been switched to an HMO (health management organization) with which the surgeon she knew and trusted was not affiliated. Much to her consternation, she was assigned to someone she did not know. Now she was angry at the new surgeon, who in her view had botched the job. The repressed anger toward her family and herself was now transferred and projected onto the surgeon. She continued to work on her mental-emotional issues and subsequently did well.

In another case, a woman had been diagnosed with vulvar cancer. She acknowledged in therapy that she had been sexually fondled by her father as a young girl and had never resolved the anger and shame she felt over the incident. Her present cancer was located right where he had touched her. After work to appropriately resolve and release her negative feelings, she initially felt much better. She was under pressure to have the cancer surgically removed as soon as possible. After surgery, she suffered an inordinate amount of pain and experienced slow wound-healing and prolonged discomfort. In addition, she believed that her surgeon had removed more tissue than he had indicated would be necessary, and so she felt violated by him and enraged. In fact, she had not completely resolved her anger toward her father nor her feelings of guilt. These feelings contributed to the complications of her surgery and were now transferred onto the surgeon. More mental and emotional work was required.

It is important when dealing with surgical and medical complications not to blame the doctor or medical staff but to face the feelings directly by taking dominion over them for healing. Medical staffs simply fulfill roles determined by our subconscious emotional energy.

The use of what I call gross energy—subatomic particulate energy (X-ray and other types of radioactive energies) and high intensity thermal energy—in the treatment of certain diseases also has predictable results. The outcome of these therapies, as discussed, will be determined by how well the recipient faces and releases negative mental and emotional dynamics. With willingness, vigilance and proper focus, potential negative side-effects can be minimized or eliminated.

One patient who had undergone a lumpectomy for removal of a breast cancer had felt intuitively that she was healed after spiritual work. But to make her doctor and family comfortable, she agreed to undergo X-ray therapy. In order to deal with her fear of this procedure's known side-effects, she used the formula. She underwent her treatments in a prayerful, meditative state, visualizing Jesus sitting with her holding her hands; and she amazed everyone with the results: absolutely no side-effects from the irradiation and no residual reduction in breast size even after a generous lumpectomy.

Pharmaceutical medicine is based on the premise that molecule-to-molecule interactions must necessarily occur for a drug to have an effect. This field evolved as the science of chemistry advanced to the point of successfully isolating and then synthesizing the active molecules of herbal remedies. It is the main modality for therapy in allopathic medicine. Molecular interactions are predictable because molecules follow the dynamic of the intent behind their manifestation. These dynamics form and follow the natural laws of this world's reality construct. They can be utilized for our benefit or for our harm depending on the nature of the dominant emotional energy of the individuals having the experience. Again, potentially harmful effects may be minimized or eliminated with willingness to love, proper vigilance and focus.

Surgical, gross energetic and molecularly mediated therapies are not the only means through which physical change can be initiated. Some energy interactions may not take place at the molecule-to-molecule level, and yet they can have effects on the molecular experience of the body. In other words, the body may receive the energy for change directly through its energy field without receiving an associated active molecular agent. Such effects cannot be explained based on molecule-to-molecule dynamics. This phenomenon is common in therapies generally referred to as alternative medicine.

Because these more subtle energy interactions cannot be readily explained within the framework of current mainstream medicine, which is limited to a molecular reality, they fall into the category of the supernatural and are thus suspect. In the past, serious effort, including the investment of funds, has not been made to investigate alternative remedies or techniques. But recently, Congress, as a result of "grass roots" experiences and pressure, has allotted a relatively small fund to the National Institutes of Health to set up an alternative medicine division.

Even if funds are made available, the design of the research may not be appropriate and could lead to more confusion because the traditional view does not recognize the role consciousness plays in affecting molecular outcome. Because energy interactions and thus molecular experience follow the dominant intent of the individual in a given situation, those who have a strong disbelief may not be successful in demonstrating through their research that what they do not believe in is actually possible. The results of research tend to reflect the faith of the researcher.

My first observation of this phenomenon occured when I was a medical student, although I did not understand then what the dynamic was. While working on research projects, I reviewed journal articles reporting basic research where the data from one laboratory clearly supported one conclusion, while data from another laboratory repeating the studies supported the opposite conclusion. Who was in error? In some cases the data was so clear for each opposing view that we might conclude that one of the parties was intellectually dishonest. Actually both parties may have been right. The results of research tend to follow the intent of the researchers if their point of view and desire is strongly held. Each laboratory got the results it had faith in. It is the nature of our scientific community to be skeptical and competitive, so it isn't uncommon for one group to have a vested interest in proving the other group wrong.

In the case of homeopathic remedies and flower essences, there is no molecular basis for explaining their effect. They operate at a prephysical energy level to change the molecular experience of the patient. Regarding homeopathic medicine, the initial substance of a remedy is diluted to such an extent that the final solution is not likely to contain any molecules of the substance. The molecules of the solution are not active as a remedy, but they could be thought of as the carriers of subtle energy to the patient, where it has its effect. That subtle energy, of course, is the energy of the intent of the collective consciousness of all who participate in developing and refining a particular system of therapy. In addition to the collective energy of intent already within the system, other essential ingredients are the intent and faith of both the practitioner delivering the therapy and the patient, and the integrity of their interaction.

When used for disease therapy, herbal remedies, nutritional therapies and food supplements may operate at the molecule-to-molecule level or solely at the subtle energy level, depending on the specific remedy and the situation for which it is used. Some pharmaceuticals may also be effective due to the energy of intent they carry independent of their molecular activity. The effectiveness of the interaction matches the intensity of intention and faith of the collective consciousness of the individuals involved.

Various appliances and magnetic and electromagnetic energy sources have been developed for healing. Their effectiveness also follows the energy of intent and the faith of the participants in the healing activity. It is interesting that electromagnetic energy from household and office appliances and power lines is considered by some to be hazardous. Yet in other situations electromagnetic energy is used for healing. Needless to say, more investigative work in this area, with an understanding of the involvement of consciousness as cause, would be useful.

In the case of touch therapies—such as various forms of massage, healing-touch therapies and acupressure—the energy of intent is expressed in the mechanics of touching. The most significant interaction, however, occurs between the energy field of the practitioner and the energy field of the patient. The movement of energy and its effect are expressions of the combined intent of the two. Because of their tactile nature, touch therapies have an increased ability to get the patient's attention and thus to facilitate the movement and release of blocked emotional energy.

Some forms of healing-touch therapy do not actually involve physical touch, as the practitioner works in the energy field of the patient. These could be called non-contact healing therapies. Different systems go by a variety of names. The Russians refer to them as bioenergy therapies. Although no touch is involved, the patient, if conscious, is very much aware of the therapeutic interaction

Manipulative therapies are also available. Their effectiveness may to some extent be explained by the mechanical effect they have upon the body. However, their effects are ultimately the manifestations of the intent of the participants and are not limited to problems that one would ordinarily consider musculoskeletal (mechanical) in nature.

Acupuncture is a technique of stimulating the body's energy points and energy meridians by the introduction and manipulation of needles at the these points. The mechanics of the procedure get the attention and involvement of the patient. As in all therapies, its effectiveness is a measure of the intent and faith of the participants.

The energy of intent can also be effectively administered through various rituals for healing. With the combined readiness of the patient and the faith of both patient and practitioner, these rituals can be useful tools for healing.

Simply sitting and talking with or listening to a patient while in a centered state of love with the intent to help and heal can result in appropriate energy interactions for healing. If the patient is receptive, these interactions can facilitate emotional release and physical change as effectively as any of the above-mentioned procedures. However, some people may need a remedy or procedure as a tool of faith and to help maintain their focus.

The practitioner-client, interactive healing phenomenon may also be non-local. The recipient does not have to be in the physical presence of the practitioner or even consciously aware of the activity for healing to occur if at some level the patient is ready. But again, being in the presence of the practitioner and participating directly in the process may be needed in order to enhance faith and maintain focus.

At this point in the human experience, some areas on earth have a higher energy quality and thus afford a better milieu for healing. Some of these locations are remote areas in nature that have been less affected by the negative consciousness of humankind. Other places exhibit the benefit of the positive effects of man's love and spiritual practice. Churches, monasteries, spiritual retreat centers and healing centers, particularly those with a long, positive history, can serve as sources of positive energy and therefore provide a good setting for healing.

Faith that a remedy or healing technique will have a certain effect can come about through a variety of ways. The remedy may be part of an ancient tradition or legend passed down or rediscovered. Or faith may come about because of the remedy's contextual relationship to a particular individual's experience. For example, if an individual has spontaneously released the mental and emotional equivalents of a certain disease or set of symptoms—even though he may not realize the relationship of the mind to the body's experience—he is now ready for healing. If he takes a remedy and experiences healing, he may associate great healing power with the remedy. In fact, however, the remedy served as a tool of faith. Although he was ready to get well, he needed something that seemed to be outside himself to satisfy his belief system and therefore to effect a cure. As a result of his experience, his faith in the remedy is strengthened.

Let us suppose that he is inspired by his experience and, in his enthusiasm, wants to share the remedy with others. If he has released enough repressed anger and guilt, he will not sabotage his intent;

instead, he will attract others who are ready to get well but also need a tool of faith. With positive results, the discoverer's faith increases, and the new recipient's faith adds the collective energy of intent. Still others receive the remedy and have positive results. Enthusiasm extends beyond a few selective conditions for which the remedy has been successful in the past, and it is tried for other diseases or symptoms. Because of the growing collective faith, it is found to work there as well. Now it seems to be some sort of panacea.

But what happens if the remedy becomes so well known that it attracts people who are consciously groping for a cure for some physical problem but who have not yet released the unrecognized mental-emotional equivalents that manifested the problem? They try the remedy, and it doesn't work. Word spreads, and doubt spreads. Now the remedy becomes less effective, and there are more failures.

Let us suppose that the remedy in question is an herbal combination, although it could be any type of therapy, without a known molecular explanation for its effectiveness. Along comes a scientific critic who "knows" there is no molecular basis for the remedy's success in such a variety of conditions. He assumes that the remedy's discoverer, who is perhaps now marketing it, is simply a greedy con artist. The critic obtains funds and sets up a scientific study to debunk the fraudulent remedy and protect the public. Because of his intent, he unconsciously attracts participants who are not ready to get well. And this combination—his lack of faith and blocked participants—results in failure. The results are publicized. Now the remedy becomes generally less effective. What could have been a harmless and beneficial tool of faith with a strong energy of intent for healing is now gone. How the discoverer of the remedy fares in all this depends on his vigilance and focus.

Now let us suppose that a remedy is introduced by someone who truly intends to defraud and who has no faith in his product. Perhaps he has paid people to give false testimony in order to market it. In this situation, some people may actually have positive results because of the strength of their own intent and faith in the remedy, in spite of the lack of faith of its producer and distributor.

A remedy, of course, will be much more powerful and more effective when all participants are focused in faith on a common intent. In the early days of medicine, the physician would hand the medication to the patient with the intent that it have a certain effect. Today the patient frequently goes to someone other than the prescribing physician to get the prescription filled. That person may not be as involved or as focused on the common intent, and the potential of increasing its effectiveness may be lost. But in fact the prescribing practitioner does not have to be physically involved with the remedy for his intent to be associated with it. However, as is frequently the case, he may tend to be distracted; so his physical involvement, such as in its distribution, may help him maintain focus on the intent.

Doctors today are trained to be skeptics and to warn patients of the worst possible scenarios so as not to give false hope and cause disappointment. This tendency dilutes the energy of intent and weakens faith, which tends to decrease the effectiveness of the therapy. I agree with the statement made by Bernie Siegel, M.D., in one of his talks, "There is no such thing as false hope."[104, 105, 106]

It is not the purpose of this chapter to give a detailed discussion of alternative medicine. More detailed information can be found in the books *Vibrational Medicine* by Richard Gerber, M.D.,[32] and *Energetic Healing* by James Eden, M.D.[24] For those looking for assistance from these alternative areas, observe the experience of others. If a system has worked for many people, you can assume that it has a lot of energy of intent behind it into which you can tap, and to which you can add your own intent. If willingness is present, healing can occur in this way.

Of course, it is possible to simply reach for the faith that you are well while expressing a willingness to love unconditionally, and to accept healing as a direct energetic experience from within. However, to insist that healing must come in this way when it may be easier for us, because of our level of faith, to use a remedy, is a symptom of spiritual pride. Such insistence is an attempt to struggle against and conquer guilt rather than transcend it.

Because of our inability to believe in the direct presence of God acting in ourselves, we may still need to put our faith in something that seems to be outside of self. Love operates within the limits of our belief system to maintain our peace and comfort; sometimes it actually manipulates circumstances to increase that faith and enhance receptivity. Linda, a friend of mine, related such an incident. She spent three months in India visiting Sai Baba (Chapter 5, p. 41). Although she had several interviews with him, she never had the opportunity to tell him about her brother, who had cancer. When it came time to leave, she realized that her chance was gone. In tears while packing, she heard a knock on her door. It was one of Sai Baba's volunteers carrying a paper bag. "This is for your brother," he said. "Sai Baba said for him to take it." Inside the bag were twelve small old newspaper packets filled with vibhuti, the ash Sai Baba frequently materializes and gives to many who come to see him as a symbolic expression of love. She was overjoyed. Sai Baba had known about her brother and had provided for him.

Linda arrived home in the States late in the evening. After the fanfare of an excited reunion with her family, including her ailing brother, she went to bed. She awoke early the next morning in a state of concern. She had placed the bag of vibhuti on the kitchen counter the previous evening and in the excitement of her return had forgotten about it. She rushed down to the kitchen to see if it was still there. She knew that it would be unlikely that anyone would have recognized its significance, and it might have been mistaken for trash. Sure enough, it was gone. She checked the garbage, but it had already been picked up. Her brother was now up. Linda explained the situation. Yes, he had seen the bag and had himself placed it in the garbage. In distress, she went back to bed. As she lay there crying, it dawned on her to pray about the situation. As she was praying, her nephew opened the door to her room and said, "Here Aunt Linda. Look what I found on the shelf in my room." There it was: the intact bag of vibuhti—neither crushed nor stained by garbage. The bag and its contents had apparently materialized in her nephew's room. No one in the house had retreived it. Overjoyed, she took it to her brother. He was an engineer, limited to a molecular view of reality, and under ordinary circumstances would never have done something as ridiculous as swallow ash to cure cancer or have the faith that would have allowed a cure to occur had he taken it. But now things were different. He had personally thrown away the bag, but here it was again. He took the ash as directed, and he had no more problem with cancer. In addition, the nephew developed a stronger interest in spirituality.

Experiences such as these demonstrate the powerful, ongoing dynamic of the energy of loving intent. I have a friend who was dragged to see Sai Baba by his wife while on a business trip in India. Al had little interest in spirituality and no interest in Sai Baba, but being fairly patient he agreed to accompany her on what he considered silly side trips. One such trip before visiting Sai Baba was to a small temple that had been blessed by him. The temple priest lifted a coin-sized medallion out of a cup of liquid, dried it off and placed it in Al's hand. To his amazement, beads of liquid welled up on the surface of the metal, filling and overflowing the palm of his hand. He could not deny what he was seeing. He was being introduced to a new paradigm. The priest explained that when Sai Baba had blessed the temple, he had also materialized the medallion and instructed the priest to place it in a cup. Ever since, the medallion has been producing a tasty nectar that fills the cup.

This is a graphic demonstration of the power of the energy of intent when the mind initiating the thought is completely unified with the thought, free of the energies of fear and doubt—in other words, when the mind comes from pure love and total faith. Al went on to an encounter with Sai Baba that was very rewarding and instructive. His experiences brought about changes in perception for him and a new approach to life, leading to higher states of peace and joy.

As we focus on love and learn to live more spontaneously in the moment, without judgment, the intuitive wisdom of love will guide us to the best therapies. One patient had developed cardiac arrhythmias that were causing symptoms. She had intuitively found that by eating salt she could control the arrhythmias. This occurred before her laboratory workup revealed a salt-losing nephropathy, which is a kidney condition that causes loss of salt in the urine and seriously low levels of salt in the body.

Another patient was guided to use visualization. She had developed a thyroid tumor. On palpatation it was very firm, which is typical for a carcinoma of the thyroid gland. However, we never got a tissue diagnosis, because the tumor disappeared in sixteen days. Although I was seeing her as a pathologist to do the thyroid scan and not as her primary physician or therapist, she had heard one of my talks and knew the formula. After praying for healing she developed a compulsion to visualize the surgical removal of the tumor. This was appropriate for her because she was an operating room nurse and had assisted in many such procedures. In her imagination—over and over again for sixteen days—she saw herself undergoing pre-operative preparation, going through surgery, in recovery, and even having the sutures removed. Even if the tumor had not been malignant, it would not have been likely that a benign tumor including a cyst would have resolved in such a short period of time under usual circumstances.

Although various therapies and remedies directed at the body are useful because of one's cultural belief system, all healing occurs at the level of the mind and involves the need for changing perceptions and releasing negative emotional energy. To ignore this and to focus only on the body or some external situation results in delay and more confusion. Approaches to mental healing such as cognitive counseling, intuitive counseling, dream interpretation and the induction of altered states of consciousness (including guided meditation and visualization, hypnosis and various types of breath work) are all useful in uncovering and releasing negative emotions and in opening oneself to new perceptions.

In the final analysis, life itself with all its events is an ongoing workshop for the purpose of healing. All we need do is to focus on love in every moment and in every situation. Love heals all. If we have trouble focusing, the tools mentioned above may be useful. Working with a loving facilitator, no matter which technique is used, increases the healing energy as compared to working alone. Joining with other minds in common purpose exponentially increases the energy of intent.

What I have said in earlier discussions of remedies also applies to diet. As we learn to live more spontaneously and to focus on love, intuitive wisdom will guide us to the best foods. In other words, if we approach the universe with love, our eating habits will reflect that love. One thing we will want to do is give up eating the flesh of animals. If you have ever visited a slaughterhouse, you know that what happens there is not loving. Our goal is for the world to become a reflection of, and a metaphor for, love. Animals raised for food are treated as objects without feelings—in other words, cruelly. As they approach slaughter, they suffer a great deal of fear and anger, which are obvious to the observer. I once talked with the CEO of a grocery chain. He said that after a visit to a slaughterhouse, it bothered him that he had to sell meat.

The fear and anger of the animal is not without effect on its flesh, which becomes our food. At the molecular level, this is seen in the increase in sympathomimetic molecules—the molecules of stress such as epinephrine and nor-epinephrine—in the tissue fluids of the meat. At a more subtle level, the energy field of the meat takes on the vibration of fear and anger, which we assimilate into our own energy fields as we eat the meat.

The effect is seen in problems that are more common in meat eaters such as carcinoma of the colon and cardiovascular disease. At the mental level, the mood is affected by a subtle or not-so-subtle increase in the level of worry and irritability. In someone who has been on a meat diet all his or her life, this will not be noticeable. Considering where our perceptions are as a culture, there is plenty that seems to justify our worry and irritability. In someone who has been a non-meat eater for a long period of time, it would be noticeable if he or she were to go back to a meat diet. In addition to the negative energy we absorb by eating meat, at some level in the deep unconscious we "know" this is not loving. There will be repressed guilt, although not justified, related to the killing of the animals, and at some point the guilt must be dealt with.

Furthermore, our bodies are not made to eat meat. Humans have a gastrointestinal tract almost exactly like that of a gorilla, a strong, four-hundred-pound vegetarian. Heavy meat diets result in increased intraluminal pressure in the colon, causing diverticulosis, which may evolve into diverticulitis. The increased transit time through the intestinal tract caused by a heavy meat diet may result in increased exposure to potentially toxic materials, including carcinogens that may be in the food.

However, we should not condemn those who eat meat. As individuals and as cultures we do the best we can based on past experiences of scarcity, which caused us to turn to the flesh of animals for food.

And we also need to bear in mind that for animals as well as humans, slaughter is an experience, not reality.

In my own experience, I was healed of arthritis without any change in diet. Like most of us, I was raised on a meat diet. During and immediately after my physical healing, I ate meat as well as the usual quantity of highly processed foods common to the American diet. Love transcended any negative effect of the food. Later I changed my diet, not primarily for health reasons, but as an expression of the sensitivity and compassion of love. I first gave up all mammalian meat, and later fowl flesh. Ultimately I will give up fish and other seafood. After my conscious choice to give up meat I was given specific dietary advice: eat vegetables primarily, raw whenever possible or cooked as little as possible, and eat dairy products and seafood in moderation.

The intuitive and mystical information that guided me was that cows, pigs and other mammals have an energy of consciousness as do humans. This consciousness incarnates in the body and experiences the world through it just as we do. It also has an emotional and social experience unique to its species. In most cases, the mammal does not give of itself voluntarily to be eaten but instead feels as you would if you were rounded up to be slaughtered. Although the experience is not the reality of the animal—for in reality the animal is not a body, just as you and I are not—it is not the best way to teach love. For the animal, it is a nightmare.

The consciousness that manifests lower animals such as fish and perhaps some fowl is not incarnate in the animal and knows it is not the animal. This is similar to the situation for plants. The lower animals are instinctual in that they have been programmed to survive. Thus the fish on a line attempts to get away, but it has no emotional experience related to being caught. What is taken with gratitude may be given with gratitude—for instance, the salmon swimming upstream to spawn. She lays her eggs and dies, leaving her dead body to nourish the newly hatched fish.

Generally speaking, foods that are as close to nature as possible or that are raised and handled by people consciously focused on the intent to love will be the most helpful and healthy. When man attempts to improve food and food productivity while focused on ego needs instead of love, the outcome will be compromised by the fear and guilt that motivate the ego's desire. The outcome will be less than optimal and may even be detrimental. Food handled by anxious, irritated people begins to take on that emotional vibration, which will have to be dealt with by the one consuming the food. In other words, food handled by people with mental indigestion may cause physical indigestion. Thus, because of the state of consciousness of humankind, highly processed foods are usually not the most beneficial.

In the realm of food production, the use of insecticides and chemical fertilizers has disrupted the natural process of production and assimilation of plant nutrients, and left behind toxic residues. This practice also has a negative impact on the soil's capacity to replenish itself, thus creating dependency on continued use of chemical fertilizers.

There is a way to commune with nature so that we interact most productively and joyously with our environment.[28, 131] When we choose to work and interact with nature with love as our conscious intent, we will intuitively be led to the most helpful actions.

This is not to say that all processed foods or even highly processed or synthetic remedies are harmful. If the food is processed or the remedy synthesized with loving intent, the result can be just as beneficial, or even more so, than the natural or unprocessed product.

Back to the subject of animals, I don't mean to say that the act of eating mammalian flesh is always unloving. There have been occasions when an animal has allowed itself to be killed to give sustenance to someone in need. This is an act of love on the part of the animal. The native cultures offered prayers of apology and gratitude to the souls of animals and took only what they needed. Blessing the food in prayer and receiving it with love and gratitude will assist in transmuting its negative energy. Still, the practice of eating animal flesh is not the ultimate metaphor for truth. It is important now to allow our culture to embrace the idea that scarcity and animal sacrifice to provide food are not necessary.

There are those who argue that animals eat each other, and since God created the animals this way, it must be all right for us to eat them as well. The evolution of animals has not followed the will of God. Evolution of species where the strong hunt and eat the weak is not a reflection of love but a manifestation of the belief in scarcity and the collective fear and anger of humankind, and then, ultimately, animalkind. The collective animal consciousness, or animal kingdom, was created with an inherent responsiveness to the thoughts and feelings of man (again, the dominion of man referred to in the Bible). Much of the animal kingdom followed the human fall in consciousness. If human consciousness had not fallen into fear and guilt, the human-to-animal and animal-to-animal relationships would have remained a loving and creative experience. When humankind regains its senses, we will return to that state.

Some of my statements about the suffering of animals may seem strong and guilt-inducing, but that is not my intent. Meat eaters are not to be condemned. Members of my family still eat meat, and it is served in my home on occasion. It is not useful to force people to give up a meat diet before they are ready. As for the animals' experience, as I have said, it is an unhappy experience but not their reality. Guilt is not appropriate.

This brings us to a discussion of appropriate empathy. The world as a lower-dimensional experience is equivalent to an illusion or dream. It is not reality. To react to it as reality continues the illusion, because our emotions continue to determine our outer experience, and the future becomes a reflection of the past—a reflection of our emotions. Both animals and humans are experiencing much suffering in the world of today. If we insist on reacting to the suffering of others as their reality and accept sadness, we will accentuate their experience of sadness and add to the collective sadness of the planet. But our role is not to ignore the pain of others. We do realize they are in pain and appropriately desire to help them become free of it. To be most helpful, we must not allow another's pain to become our pain even as the love and joy of God in us causes us to reach out with wise assistance. If we follow this course, the experience of suffering will eventually end for everyone, and all consciousness will return to the peace of God. Free will gives us the choice of when, not whether. We can appropriately influence the choices of others, but we cannot make them for others. To attempt to do so usually results in delay and more pain. Through the use of the healing formula we can maintain our peace in a world of suffering without judgment, condemnation, guilt or grief. It is useful to think of and visualize the sufferer as whole and complete. Such thoughts and their emotional energy will influence and help in the manifestation and experience of wholeness.

Chapter 16

TOWARD REALITY

There is much in nature that represents the "mis-creation" of mankind. The energy of collective consciousness manifests itself through the unconscious out-picturing of its content in the physical experience. The negative things of the world are the monsters in our collective dream. However, if properly recognized, they are not negative at all but opportunities for bringing up repressed emotions for healing. Energy, in a sense, is entrapped in negative images and events by the effect of our collective misthinking. These negative aspects of nature warrant our love for their healing and release. Because they exist in our consciousness, our love and patience for them is actually our love and patience for ourselves. Thus things like mosquitos, ticks, fleas, ferocious animals, poison ivy, pathogenic bacteria, viruses, parasites, and destructive storms, earth movements, forest fires and floods need love and patience even as we deal with them appropriately, so that we don't experience suffering. To kill a flea may be seen as an act of love that allows negative energy trapped in the form of a flea to be transformed. As a lower animal, the flea is an instinctual being—the equivalent of a biologically computerized robot of torment.

As the collective consciousness of the planet changes, we will continue to see changes in nature. Some of these changes may appear calamitous if we resist the higher energy of love that is now healing fear in the planet. However, these calamitous changes are the manifestations of the release of negative energy, and this release will ultimately yield positive results. As we focus on love, we will ride through these events in safety.

If we live practicing the formula, focusing on love in the moment, we will become impermeable to negative energies, even those appearing as molecular and physical interactions. The power of love, which is not limited by the past or by natural laws, will transcend them even to the point of altering the continuity of linear time. Events considered supernatural or miraculous will be commonly observed. Tumors will disappear, instant physical changes will occur, the body will become immune to toxins or noxious physical agents (for example, even the effect of fire). The body will also become less dependent on sleep, food or certain nutrients that have been considered essential. Also the environment and events around us will change, bringing about the experience of safety and peace. Imagine a world without fear, guilt, anger and their effects—a world without poverty, struggle, conflict, disease and death.

Is it possible to reprogram the body so that it does not degenerate and die, so that it maintains youth and vitality as long as we have need of it? The answer is yes. Although for many this answer is unbelievable, such a reality is not beyond the concepts of modern physics and the cutting edge of biological science. Traditional science has described the evolution of the species as a process of "natural" selection and adaptation to a changing environment. This process had to involve genetic mutations that are believed to have been random events resulting in this natural selection and bringing about changes in the biology and structure of organisms. However, these changes were not the result of random selection but the effect of consciousness. In the future, as consciousness changes, DNA structure and function will also change, producing new genetic codes and altering cellular function. The body will change. In the animal kingdom this includes changes in species. As the Bible predicts, "The wolf will live with the lamb, the leopard will lie down with the goat, the calf and the lion and the yearlings together and the child shall lead them. The cow will feed with the bear and their young lie down together, and the lion will eat straw like the ox" (Isaiah 11:6-7). Some species may seem to disappear, and new species will appear.

In regards to humankind, in the next few decades those who become spiritually open will experience a tremendous increase in life expectancy. This life extension will not be the result of technology but of a change in human consciousness and in the energy field that makes the body. Such change will not require aeons of time. For those who choose to follow the healing formula, change is available now.

Would the world become overpopulated if we could live in body as long as we desire? Actually the world could support many more than the current five billion people in peace, health and prosperity if everyone lived from higher consciousness. Scarcity and struggle begin with the individual and are spread as a collective experience. They are not caused by physical circumstances; physical circumstances are an effect of consciousness. Ultimately, however, once higher levels of enlightenment are experienced, it will not be our choice to live in space and time on the earth plane beyond the loving usefulness of the experience. We will choose quite naturally to return to the reality of higher dimension.

When we reach that level of enlightenment, how do we leave our current existence? The answer is: any way we choose, any way that will be the most loving for our particular circumstance. Some might let the sick body die. Others might go to sleep in a healthy body and leave during sleep. It is also possible to go into a state of meditation and eject from the body, leaving it behind. Another way to leave that serves as the ultimate metaphor for our immortality is to ascend. In this process, the energy that manifests the body is caused to rise in frequency. The body disappears from the dimension of its original frequency to reappear in a higher dimensional state or to be stored in a formless energy state. At this level of evolution, consciousness can teleport the body from place to place within the dimension of space and time, as well as inter-dimensionally. It can disappear from one place and reappear in another, to be used to communicate love. This is the ascension process that Jesus and others experienced. Jesus had the experience publicly in order to set an example for all of us. As he is recorded to have said, "He who has faith in me will do what I have been doing. He will do even greater things than these . . ." (John 14:12).

How do we reach this level of experience? By releasing the need to have the experience. As I alluded to earlier, to focus on these types of phenomena as a goal and not on the love that manifests them is to slip into attachment and spiritual pride. Love will operate in its own wisdom to bring about the changes that witness to its presence in a way most appropriate for the situation. Just follow the formula.

Appendix

MORE ON MYSTICAL AND OTHERWISE SIGNIFICANT WRITINGS

After my initial encounter with the Shroud of Turin in the spring of 1982 (see Chapter 4), the Bible[43, 96] was my main mystical reference for guiding my decisions. But two years later I still had some unanswered questions. One day while driving to work I started praying aloud with great intensity asking for an answer. Then an amazing thing happened. My prayer was interrupted in mid-sentence by a voice in my head that said: "I have given you the answer, in the life I lived and the teachings I left." And that was it. I knew the voice was from Jesus and felt overjoyed to have consciously experienced such direct communication; yet I still felt frustrated because I had been studying his teachings and hadn't found all the answers.

Shortly after this experience I was browsing through my favorite bookstore, which is noted for its collection of mystical writings, when I spotted a three-volume set of dark-blue books entitled *A Course in Miracles*.[17] I had never heard of them before, but something in me said I was to have them. I began reading the first volume, which is called "Text." It was written using Christian terminology with which I was familiar and comfortable. I recognized that it was meant to be an in-depth description of what reality is and is not, and the preface claimed that the material had been dictated by Jesus. Within a week I laid it aside. I thought that it was saying some strange things and was uncertain of its validity. I decided it was not for me.

Shortly after my dismissal of this material another synchronicity occurred. I received a letter from someone I had met briefly at a meeting. In the letter he stated that he had meant to tell me about *A Course in Miracles* and that he thought I should read it. He also enclosed a statement made by Paul as recorded in 1 Thessalonians about prophetic material: "Do not put out the Spirit's fire; do not treat prophecies with contempt. Test everything. Hold on to the good" (1 Thess. 5:20-21). I realized that the test was whether or not it was loving. And how would I tell? By its fruits.

I picked up the Course again and also began to read articles and books about its history and about people who had worked with it.* I also went to workshops and met people who were working with it. What the Course was saying was in some ways different from an orthodox or molecular view of reality, but it was the most loving thing I had ever read. It said among other things that we are innocent, that there is nothing to fear, that there is a solution to all our problems that is so wise that no one loses, and that miracles are natural and there is no order of difficulty in them. Its fruits were witnessed to by those who wrote and talked about their desperate experiences prior to finding the Course and the remarkable healing that followed as they applied what it taught. It seemed to have passed the test.

I read the 622-page text in three months and again in the following three months. I realized I was being given the long-sought-after answer to the ultimate question, "Who are we?" in the most clear, literal and blunt form yet. I was being liberated. It took me two years to complete the 478-page second volume, which is entitled "Workbook," and is formatted as lessons, one for each day. Early on I also read the

---

*References: 45, 46, 47, 108, 109, 113, 124.

88-page third volume, which is entitled "Teacher's Manual." There are also two small supplements to *A Course in Miracles—The Song of Prayer: Prayer, Forgiveness Healing*[111] and *Psychotherapy: Process and Practice.*[90]

The writing of *A Course in Miracles* began in 1966 after two clinical psychologists at Columbia University's College for Physicians and Surgeons in New York surrendered to look for a better way. Their department was in turmoil. Those who had studied the psychodynamics of consciousness had not found answers that would allow them to get along with each other. In desperation, Bill Thetford, the head of the department, gave a lamenting speech to his associate, Helen Schucman, and concluded that there must be a better way. To his surprise, Helen, who was often his adversary, agreed and said she would help him find it. Helen, Jewish by birth and atheist by choice, had a very traditional, non-mystical view of reality. Thus when she began, shortly after this declaration of intent, to have paranormal experiences, she thought she might be psychotic. She confided in Bill, who knew she was not insane. With his support they consulted experts on paranormal phenomena who were able to convince her of the validity of her experiences. One of the things she was experiencing was an inner voice interjecting itself into her awareness during undistracted moments. The voice kept saying, "This is a course in miracles, please take notes." With Bill's collaboration and support, over the next seven years she scribed *A Course in Miracles*. At one point the voice identified itself as Jesus. After my experience with the material, I had no doubt that it was. Bill immediately began to secretly apply the principles in his relationships with the members of his department. Within a year the department was transformed. I had a similar experience when I applied the information where I was working at that time.

As I mentioned, the Course uses Christian terminology. Some people have trouble with that. The reason that it was so written was to correct erroneous concepts that have permeated Christianity. For those whom this offends, the use of that terminology serves as an opportunity to forgive Christianity for all the unhappiness the ego has propagated in its name. If there is anything left unforgiven, we will be drawn to it until forgiveness is complete. Others have trouble with the use of male pronouns and nouns in reference to God, the Son of God, the Holy Spirit and mankind. This is a continuation of the traditional usage of that language by our culture generally and by early Christianity particularly. Again, for those whom it offends, it provides an opportunity to forgive. Furthermore, to have changed the language would have suggested that it made a difference, that the value of women is determined by words. In this case, to resist the error would be to make the error real and teach that the female is so weak she can be affected by the use of a pronoun.

After the second reading of the text, I "stumbled" onto a second book with the unusual title of *The Aquarian Gospel of Jesus the Christ*.[23] With the understanding given to me by my study of the Course, it was easier to accept the validity of this material, which is a good companion book to the Course. *The Aquarian Gospel* is a writing from a universal inner knowing depicting the life of Jesus, including those years skipped in the Bible. It, too, is freeing and uplifting. It came as a prophetic writing through the mind of Levi Dowling, a physician and Presbyterian minister in the mid to late 19th century. In a vision that he received on three occasions he was told that he was to "build a white city." That "white city" was *The Aquarian Gospel*, which he scribed during the quiet time of the early morning hours of two to six. Its message is the same as *A Course In Miracles*. The difference is that the Course is by Jesus in the first person, and *The Aquarian Gospel* is about Jesus in the third person.

I now felt that I had the most complete and literal teachings of Jesus and the most complete description of his life. In these teachings,

I found the answer to the question that had motivated me to pray with such intensity a year earlier. While reading this material, I reflected on the statements by Jesus found in the Bible, that I referred to in Chapter 12: "I have much more to say to you, more than you can now bear. But when he, the Spirit of truth, comes, he will guide you into all truth" (John 16:22-13). And, "Though I have been speaking figuratively, a time is coming when I will no longer use this kind of language but will tell you plainly about my Father" (John 16:25). I realized that we now had on the planet the more literal message, which because of information from modern psychology and physics we could now more readily understand.

About this time, I also discovered *The Gnostic Gospels*,[73, 95] discussed briefly in Chapter 12. This material had laid hidden in the Nag Hammadi cliffs of Egypt since the orthodox persecution of the Gnostic Christians in the fourth century, only to be rediscovered in 1945 and translated into English in 1975, the same year the Course was published. As I studied this material, I realized there were some Christians during the time of Jesus and during the early years of Christianity who were able to better understand his teachings.

Of course, there were other books besides the Bible before I found *A Course in Miracles*, *The Aquarian Gospel of Jesus the Christ* and *The Gnostic Gospels*, and others afterwards that I found useful in my journey. Some I refer to in the text of this book, and some I will mention for the first time. I was alerted to a couple of them back in my college days before I ended my conscious spiritual search in frustration and long before I resumed it as a result of my illness. While a sophomore in undergraduate school I read an article in *Time* magazine about a well-known Washington columnist who had discovered that she had a gift of automatic writing and was being given much information from other dimensions about the pre-recorded history of the earth and the nature of the earth and higher dimensions. I remember being intrigued and feeling a great desire to read this information. But I did nothing, as I was distracted by the more immediate demands of college life. About the same time I read in my Phi Gamma Delta magazine about a fraternity brother who in 1943 had died and had lived to tell about it. Again I felt intrigued and desired to know more. But again I did nothing. However, I never forgot those brief encounters. As I now reflect on them, I have the sense that my strong feelings then were the result of an intuitive connection to potential future events.

Twenty-four years later, after my physical healing and well into my compulsive spiritual search, I went into a large, well-known book store to get a particular book. Which one, I don't remember, because I did not get it. Instead, my eyes fell upon a series of books by Ruth Montgomery.[59-64] I didn't remember having ever heard of her or the books, but I felt compelled to get them. As I began reading them and about the author, I realized that she was the Washington columnist I had read about as a college sophomore. I found this material very helpful in the early stages of my search.

The same year, a new friend asked me if I had heard of Dr. George Ritchie and his book *Return From Tomorrow*.[94] I thought that I had not, so she explained that he had died in 1943 but returned to life to become a medical doctor and then a psychiatrist, and in 1972 had published a book about his experience. I got the book, and as I was reading it, I realized that Ritchie was the person I had read about in the Phi Gam magazine. When I discovered that he lived and practiced in Richmond, this time I didn't delay. I called him immediately and began to work with him on my spiritual search. He pointed out to me the writings of Emmet Fox[30] and Starr Daily,[18] both of which were very useful. Daily's book *Release* gave me a clearer and more practical understanding of the teachings of Jesus as recorded in the Bible. These and other books mentioned in this text, as well as some not mentioned,[27, 79] served as tools that helped me to become more open to the intuitive experience of an inner wisdom and thus better able to accept and understand the Course and other more recent material.

The Edgar Cayce center, the Association for Research and Enlightenment, is only a couple of hours from Richmond, so I took advantage of its programs and materials and found them useful. The biography of Edgar Cayce, *There Is A River*,[114] was also inspiring.

After *A Course in Miracles*, I thought I had finished my reading and was quite resistant to anything else. Another event, however, intervened. I was working with an acquaintance to help her attune to her Higher Self to understand why she was experiencing an illness. She was also helping me to attune to my Higher Self. We took turns leading each other in guided meditations. In every session she told me about the *"I AM" Discourses*,[33] which were dictated by St. Germain in a way similar to the dictation of *A Course In Miracles*. I listened patiently but had no interest. One day she handed me the book and insisted that I read the first few pages aloud to her. She would not have it any other way. To appease her I began reading. I then knew that I was to get the book and read it. And she discovered what was at the root of her illness.

I have subsequently allowed the Spirit of Truth to lead me to other material.* Of course, the bibliography to this book is not a complete list of all the helpful material available. Of particular note among those I have listed is the most recent book of Barbara Marx Hubbard, *The Book of Co-Creation: The Revelation, Our Crisis Is a Birth*.[44] (One should take note that prophetic utterances that are predictive in nature are the readings of the most likely future based on the dominant energy of collective consciousness at any given time. As humankind exercises free will and responds to inspiration, negative prophecies may remain unfulfilled, to be replaced by the grace of God. As more people use the formula, much negativity will be averted, both individually and collectively.)

---

*References: 4, 11, 26, 44, 58, 78, 79-89, 120, 121, 132.

Concerning technical details of spiritual practices, one may find the book *Being A Christ* by Ann and Peter Meyer useful.[58]

In addition to the more overtly mystical writings, there also are the well-known writings of my colleagues in the medical and counseling professions such as Bernie Siegel,[104-106] Larry Dossey,[20-22] Deepak Chopra,[12-15] Norman Shealy and Carolyn Myss,[103] Andrew Weil,[126] Carl Simonton,[107] and Joan Borysenko.[7] *The Celestine Prophecy*,[91] although written as fiction, also has much accurate and useful information describing the energetic phenomena related to the psychodynamics of consciousness.

It is not inherently necessary to read any of the material listed, but you are likely to find some of it useful. Some of the references can be thought of as main courses, and others fall into the category of appetizers and desserts. *A Course in Miracles* is a main dish, and I highly recommend it. There are many other good resources available that I have not listed. You will be led to what is right for you, including your own inner knowing and visionary experiences. Be open to the spontaneity of the peaceful impulse.

Books are not a substitute for inner wisdom, but are tools to help us to focus and become conscious of that wisdom more directly—to help us remember. A few years back I had the thought, after a discussion with someone who felt the Bible was the only source of the word of God, that the word of God is not written in a book but exists everywhere. Shortly after that, I was browsing through my favorite book store when my eyes fell upon *The Gospel of the Essenes*.[35] (The Essenes were a sect of Judaism that existed at the time of Jesus, prepared for his incarnation, and were among his early followers. Their original manuscripts are held in private Vatican archives, and were first translated into English in 1937.) I felt that peaceful impulse and reached out for the book. It fell open to page 146 and I read the following words:

Seek not the law in thy scripture, for the law is Life,
Whereas the scriptures are only words.
I tell thee truly,
Moses received not his laws from God in writing,
But through the living word.
The law is living word of living God
To living prophets for living men.
In everything that is life is the law written.
It is found in the grass, in the trees,
In the river, in the mountains, in the birds of heaven,
In the forest creatures and the fishes of the sea;
But it is found chiefly in thyselves.
All living things are nearer to God
Than the scriptures which are without life.
God so made life and all living things
That they might be the everliving word
Teach the laws of the Heavenly Father
And the Earthly Mother
To the sons of men.
God wrote not the laws in the pages of books,
But in thy heart and in thy spirit.
They are in thy breath, thy blood, thy bone;
In thy flesh, thine eyes, thine ears,
And in every little part of thy body.
They are present in the air, in the water,
In the earth, in the plants, in the sunbeams,
In the depths and in the heights.
They all speak to thee
That thou mayest understand the tongue and the will
Of the living God.
The scriptures are the works of man,
But life and all its hosts are the work of God.

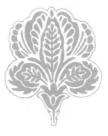

BIBLIOGRAPHY

1. Aron, Elaine, and Arthur Aron. *The Maharishi Effect: A Revolution Through Meditation. Scientific Discovery of the Astounding Power of the Group Mind.* Walpole, N.H.: Stillpoint Publishing, 1986.

2. Atwater, P.M.H. *Beyond The Light: What Isn't Being Said About Near-Death Experience.* New York: Carol Publishing Group, 1994.

3. Atwater, P.M.H. *Coming Back to Life: The After-Effects of the Near-Death Experience.* New York: Dodd, Mead & Company, 1988.

4. Bacovcin, Helen, trans. *The Way of a Pilgrim and The Pilgrim Continues His Way.* New York: Doubleday, 1978.

5. Bascam, Lionel C., and Barbara Harris. *Full Circle: The Near-Death Experience and Beyond.* New York: Pocket Books, 1990.

6. Becker, Robert O., and Gary Seldon. *The Body Electric.* New York: William Morrow and Co., 1988.

7. Borysenko, Joan. *Minding the Body and Mending the Mind.* New York: Bantam Books, 1987.

8. Brinkley, Dannion, and Paul Perry. *Saved By the Light.* New York: Villard Books, 1994.

9. Byrd, Randolph C. "Positive Therapeutic Effects of Intercessory Prayer in a Coronary Care Unit Population." *Southern Medical Journal* 81:7 (July 1988): 826-29.

10. Carothers, Merlin. *Prison to Praise.* Plainfield, N.J.: Logos International, 1979.

11. Carpenter, Tom, and Linda Carpenter. *Dialogue On Awakening:*

Communion with a Loving Brother. Princeville, Hawaii: The Carpenter Press, 1992.

12. Chopra, Deepak. *Perfect Health: The Complete Mind/Body Guide*. New York: Harmony Books, 1990.

13. Chopra, Deepak. *Quantum Healing: Exploring the Frontiers of Mind/Body Medicine*. New York: Bantam Books, 1989.

14. Chopra, Deepak. *The Seven Spiritual Laws of Success*. San Rafael, CA: Amber-Allen Publishing, 1994.

15. Chopra, Deepak. *Unconditional Life, Mastering the Forces that Shape Personal Reality*. New York: Bantam Books, 1991.

16. Clark, Ronald W. *Freud: The Man and the Cause*. New York: Random House, 1980.

17. *A Course in Miracles*. Combined Volume. Tiburon, Calif.: Foundation for Inner Peace, 1992 (original ed. 1975).

18. Daily, Starr. *Release*. New York and London: Harper & Brothers, 1942.

19. Davies, Paul. *God and the New Physics*. New York: Simon and Schuster, 1983.

20. Dossey, Larry. *Healing Words*. New York: Harper Collins Publishers, 1993.

21. Dossey, Larry. *Meaning and Medicine*. New York: Bantam Books, 1991.

22. Dossey, Larry. *Recovering the Soul: A Scientific and Spiritual Search*. New York: Bantam Books, 1989.

23. Dowling, Levi. *The Aquarian Gospel of Jesus the Christ*. Marina del Rey, Calif: DeVorss & Co., 1982.

24. Eden, James. *Energetic Healing: The Merging of Ancient and Modern Medical Practices*. New York: Plenum Press, 1993.

25. Einstein, Albert. *Relativity: The Special and the General Theory*. Translated by Robert W. Lawson. New York: Crown Publishers, 1961.

26. Essene, Virginia. *New Teachings for an Awakening Humanity*. Santa Clara, Calif.: S.E.E. Publishing Company, 1986.

27. Ferguson, Marilyn. *The Aquarian Conspiracy: Personal and Social Transformation in the 1980s*. Los Angeles: J.P. Tarcher, 1980.

28.   Findhorn Community. *The Findhorn Garden: Pioneering A New Vision of Man and Nature in Cooperation.* New York: Harper & Row Publishing, 1975.

29.   Fordham, Frieda. *An Introduction to Jung's Psychology.* New York: Penguin Books, 1966.

30.   Fox, Emmet. *The Sermon on the Mount.* New York: Harper & Row, 1938.

31.   Freud, Sigmund. *Beyond the Pleasure Principle.* Translated by James Strachey. New York: Bantam Books, 1954.

32.   Gerber, Richard. *Vibrational Medicine: New Choices for Healing Oursleves.* Santa Fe: Bear & Co., 1988.

33.   Saint Germain. *The "I AM" Discourses.* Schaumburg, Ill.: St. Germain Press, 1984.

34.   Glasser, R., et al. "Effects of Stress on Methyltransferase Synthesis: An Important DNA Repair Enzyme." *Health Psychology* 4, no. 5, 403-12, 1985.

35.   *The Gospel of the Essenes.* Translated by Edmund B. Szekely. Saffron-Walden, Great Britain: C.W. Daniels Co., Ltd., 1976.

36.   Haraldsson, Erlendur. *Modern Miracles, An Investigation of Psychic Phenomena Associated with Sathya Sai Baba.* New York: Ballantine Books, 1987.

37.   Harris, Barbara, and Lionel C. Bascom. *Full Circle: The Near Death Experience and Beyond.* New York: Simon and Schuster, 1990.

38.   Hawking, Stephen W. *A Brief History of Time: From the Big Bang to Black Holes.* New York: Bantam Books, 1988.

39.   Heller, Dr. John H. *Report on the Shroud of Turin.* Boston, Massachusetts: Houghton Mifflin Co., 1983.

40.   Herbert, Nick. *Quantum Reality: Beyond the New Physics.* Garden City, N.Y.: Anchor Press, 1985.

41.   Hislop, John. *My Baba and I.* Prasantha Nilayam, India: Sri Sathy Sai Books and Publication Trust, 1989.

42.   Holmes, Ernest. *The Science of Mind.* New York: Dodd, Mead and Company, 1938.

43.   *The Holy Bible. New International Version.* Grand Rapids, Mich.:

Zondervan Bible Publishers, 1978.

44.   Hubbard, Barbara Marx. *The Book of Co-Creation: The Revelation, Our Crisis Is a Birth.* Sonoma, Calif.: The Foundation for Conscious Evolution, 1993.

45.   Jampolsky, Gerald G. *Love Is Letting Go of Fear.* New York: Bantam Books, 1981.

46.   Jampolsky, Gerald G. *Teach Only Love.* New York: Bantam Books, 1983.

47.   Jampolsky, Gerald G., with Patricia Hopkins and William N. Metford. *Good Bye to Guilt: Releasing Fear Through Forgiveness.* New York: Bantam Books, 1985.

48.   Judith, Anodea. *Wheels of Life: A Natural History of the Supernatural.* St. Paul, Minn.: Llewyllyn Publications, 1989.

49.   Jung, Carl G., ed. *Man and His Symbols.* New York: Dell Publishing Co., 1982.

50.   Jung, Carl G. *Synchronicity: An Acausal Connecting Principle.* Translated by R.F.C. Hull. Princeton, N.J.: Princeton University Press, 1973.

51.   Justice, Blair. *Who Gets Sick.* Los Angeles: J. P. Tarcher, 1988.

52.   Kaku, Michio, and Jennifer Trainer. *Beyond Einstein: The Cosmic Quest for the Theory of the Universe.* New York: Bantam Books, 1987.

53.   Kiecolt-Glaser, J.K., et al. "Distress and DNA Repair in Human Lymphocytes." *Journal of Behavioral Medicine* 8, no. 8, 311-19.

54.   Kübler-Ross, Elizabeth. *On Death and Dying.* New York: Macmillan Publishing Co., 1969.

55.   Lazaris. *The Lazaris Material: The Mysterious Power of the Chakras.* Los Angeles: Concept: Synergy (Audio Tapes), 1986.

56.   McGarey, Gladys T. *Born To Live.* Phoenix: Gabriel Press, 1980.

57.   Malz, Betty. *My Glimpse of Eternity.* Grand Rapids: Chosen Books, 1978.

58.   Meyer, Ann P., and Peter V. Meyer. *Being A Christ: Inner Sensitivity Instructional Training Course.* San Diego, Calif.: Dawning Publications, 1975.

59.   Montgomery, Ruth. *Here and Hereafter.* New York: Fawcett Crest, 1968.

60.   Montgomery, Ruth. *A Search for Truth*. New York: Fawcett Crest, 1966.

61.   Montgomery, Ruth. *Strangers Among Us*. New York: Fawcett Crest, 1976.

62.   Montgomery, Ruth. *Threshold of Tomorrow*. New York: G.P. Putnam Sons, 1982.

63.   Montgomery, Ruth. *The World Before*. New York: Fawcett Crest, 1976.

64.   Montgomery, Ruth. *A World Beyond*. New York: Fawcett Crest, 1971.

65.   Moody, Raymond, Jr. *Reflections on Life After Life*. Toronto: Bantam Books, 1977.

66.   Moses, Jeffrey. *Oneness: Great Principles Shared by All Religions*. New York: Ballantine Books, 1989.

67.   Murphet, Howard. *Sai Baba: Avatar*. San Diego: Birth Day Publishing Co., 1977.

68.   Murphet, Howard. *Sai Baba: Invitation To Glory*. Madras: S.G. Wasari for Macmillan India Limited, 1989.

69.   Murphet, Howard. *Sai Baba: Man of Miracles*. Madras: Macmillan India Limited, 1988.

70.   Nordenström, Björn E. W. *Biologically Closed Electrical Circuits: Clinical, Experimental and Theoretical Evidence for an Additional Circulatory System*. Stockholm: Nordic Medical Publications, 1983.

71.   O'Connor, Peter. *Understanding Jung, Understanding Yourself*. New York: Paulist Press, 1985.

72.   Osis, Karlis, and Erlendur Haraldsson. *At the Hour of Death*. New York: Avon Books, 1977.

73.   Pagels, Elaine. *The Gnostic Gospels*. New York: Vintage Books, 1989.

74.   Pagels, Heinz R. *The Cosmic Code: Quantum Physics as the Language of Nature*. New York: Simon and Schuster, 1982.

75.   Pagels, Heinz R. *Perfect Symmetry: The Search for the Beginning of Time*. New York: Simon and Schuster, 1985.

76.   Pais, Abraham. *Subtle Is the Lord: The Science and the Life of Albert Einstein*. Oxford: Oxford University Press, 1983.

77.   Peat, F. David. *Superstrings and the Search for The Theory of Everything*.

Chicago: Contemporary Books, 1988.

78. Peck, M. Scott. *A Different Drum.* New York: Simon and Schuster, 1987.

79. Peck, M. Scott. *The Road Less Traveled.* New York: Simon and Schuster, 1978.

80. Pictor, Mike. *Conversations with Christ.* Farmingdale, N.Y.: Coleman Publishing, 1984.

81. Pierrakos, Eva. *Guide Lectures for Self-Transformation.* Phoenicia, N.Y.: Pathworks Press, 1985.

82. Pierrakos, John. *Core Energetics. Developing the Capacity to Heal.* Mendocino, Calif.: Life Rhythms Publications, 1987.

83. Price, John Randolph. *The Angels Within Us.* New York: Ballantine Books, 1993.

84. Price, John Randolph. *The Manifestation Process.* Austin, Texas: The Quartus Foundation for Spiritual Research, 1983.

85. Price, John Randolph. *The Planetary Commission.* Austin, Texas: The Quartus Foundation for Spiritual Resesarch, 1984.

86. Price, John Randolph. *Practical Spirituality.* Austin, Texas: The Quartus Foundation for Spiritual Research, 1985.

87. Price, John Randolph. *A Spiritual Philosophy for the New Work.* Boerme, Texas: Quartus Books, 1990.

88. Price, John Randolph. *The Super Beings.* Austin, Texas: The Quartus Foundation for Spiritual Research, 1981.

89. Price, John Randolph. *With Wings as Eagles.* Austin, Texas: The Quartus Foundation for Spiritual Research, 1987.

90. *Psychotherapy: Purpose, Process and Practice.* Tiburon, Calif: Foundation of Inner Peace, 1976.

91. Redfield, James. *The Celestine Prophecy.* Hoover, Ala.: Satori Publishing Co., 1993.

92. Ring, Kenneth. *Heading Toward Omega: In Search of the Meaning of the Near Death Experience.* New York: William Morrow & Co., 1984.

93. Ritchie, George G., Jr. *My Life After Dying: Becoming Alive to Universal Love.* Norfolk, Va.: Hampton Roads Publishing Co., 1991.

94. Ritchie, George G., Jr., and Elizabeth Sherrill. *Return from Tomorrow.* Grand Rapids: Chosen Books, 1978.

95. Robinson, James M., general editor. *The Nag Hammadi Library.* New York: Harper & Row Publishers, 1981 (revised ed. 1988).

96. *The Ryrie Study Bible.* New Testament. King James Version. Chicago: Moody Press, 1976.

97. Sandweiss, Samuel H. *Sai Baba: The Holy Man and The Psychiatrist.* Anantapur, India: Sri Sathya Sai Books and Publications Trust, 1975.

98. Sandweiss, Samuel H. *Spirit and the Mind.* Anantapur, India: Sri Sathya Sai Books and Publications Trust, 1975.

99. Schmidt, H. "Addition Effect for PK on Pre-recorded Targets." *Journal of Parapsychology* 49 (1985): 229-44.

100. Schmidt, H. "Can An Effect Precede Its Cause?" *Foundations of Physics* 8 (1981): 463-80.

101. Schmidt, H. "PK Effect on Pre-recorded Targets." *Journal of the American Society for Psychical Research* 70 (1960): 267-91.

102. Schmidt, H. "The Strange Properties of Psychokineses." *Journal of Scientific Exploration* I, no. 2 (1987): 103-18.

103. Shealy, C. Norman, and Caroline M. Myss. *The Creation of Health: Merging Traditional Medicine with Intuitive Diagnosis.* Walpole, N.H.: Stillpoint Publishing, 1988.

104. Siegel, Bernie S. *How To Live Between Office Visits.* New York: Harper Collins Publishers, 1993.

105. Siegel, Bernie S. *Love, Medicine and Miracles.* New York: Harper Collins Publishers, 1986.

106. Siegel, Bernie S. *Peace, Love and Healing.* New York: Harper Collins Publishers, 1989.

107. Simonton, O. Carl, and Reid Henson. *The Healing Journey: Restoring Health and Harmony to Body, Mind, and Spirit.* New York: Bantam Books, 1992.

108. Skutch, Judy. *Fear Binds the World.* Virginia Beach: A.R.E. Tapes, Edgar Cayce Foundation, 1983.

109. Skutch, Robert. *Journey Without Distance: The Story Behind A Course In*

Miracles. Berkeley: Celestial Arts, 1984.

110. Smith, Huston. *The World's Religions*. New York: Harper Collins Publishers, 1991.

111. *The Song of Prayer: Prayer, Forgiveness, Healing*. Tiburon, Calif.: Foundation for Inner Peace, 1978.

112. Spangler, David. *The Laws of Manifestation*. Findhorn, Scotland: Findhorn Publications, 1976.

113. *The Story of A Course In Miracles*. Videotape. Tiburon, Calif.: Foundation for Inner Peace, 1987.

114. Sugrue, Thomas. *There Is A River: The Story of Edgar Cayce*. Virginia Beach: A.R.E. Press, Edgar Cayce Foundation, 1942.

115. Talbot, Michael. *Beyond the Quantum*. New York: Macmillan Publishing Company, 1986.

116. Talbot, Michael. *The Holographic Universe*. New York: Harper Collins Publishers, 1991.

117. Tansley, David V. *Subtle Body, Essence and Shadow*. New York: Thames and Hudson, 1984.

118. Tribbe, Frank C. *Portrait of Jesus?* Briarcliff Manor, N.Y.: Stein and Day, 1983.

119. *The Upanishads*. Translated by Alistair Shearer and Peter Russell. London: Unwin Hyman Limited, 1978.

120. Valentine, Ann, and Virginia Essene. *Cosmic Revelation*. Santa Clara, Calif.: S.E.E. Publishing Co., 1987.

121. Valentine, Ann, and Virginia Essene. *Descent of the Dove*. Santa Clara, Calif.: S.E.E. Publishing Co., 1988.

122. Wald, Robert M. *Space, Time and Gravity: The Theory of the Big Bang and Black Holes*. Chicago: The University of Chicago Press, Ltd., 1977.

123. Wambach, Helen. *Life Before Life*. New York: Bantam Books, 1981.

124. Wapwich, Kenneth. *Forgiveness and Jesus*. Roscoe, N.Y.: Foundation for A Course in Miracles, 1983.

125. Watson, Lyall. *Beyond Supernature*. New York: Bantam Books, 1987.

126. Weil, Andrew. *Spontaneous Healing.* New York: Alfred A. Knopf, 1995.

127. Wilber, Ken. *Quantum Questions: Mystical Writings of the World's Great Physicists.* Boston: Shambhala Publications, 1984.

128. Wolf, Fred Alan. *Parallel Universes: The Search for Other Worlds.* New York: Simon and Schuster, 1988.

129. Wolf, Fred Alan. *Star Wave: Mind, Consciousness and Quantum Physics.* New York: Macmillan Publishing Co., 1984.

130. Wolf, Fred Alan. *Taking the Quantum Leap.* New York: Harper & Row Publishers, 1989.

131. Wright, Machaelle Small. *Behaving As If the God in All Life Mattered.* Jeffersonton, Va.: Perelandra Ltd., 1987.

132. Yogananda. *Autobiography of a Yogi.* Los Angeles: Self-Realization Fellowship, 1946.

133. Zukav, Gary. *The Dancing Wu Li Masters: An Overview of the New Physics.* New York: William Morrow and Company, 1979.